Clinical Handbook for Hospital Nurses

Clinical Handbook for Hospital Nurses

edited by

Ann Close and George Castledine

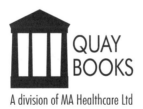

QUAY
BOOKS

A division of MA Healthcare Ltd

Quay Books Division, MA Healthcare Ltd, St Jude's Church, Dulwich Road,
London SE24 0PB

British Library Cataloguing-in-Publication Data
A catalogue record is available for this book

Printed in the UK by Bath Press, Lower Bristol Road, Bath, BA2 3BL

Contents

List of contributors

Editors

Ann Close, Nursing Director, The Dudley Group of Hospitals NHS Trust and

George Castledine, Professor of Nursing, The University of Central England and The Dudley Group of Hospitals NHS Trust

Chapter Contributors

George Castledine, Professor of Nursing The University of Central England and The Dudley Group of Hospitals NHS Trust

Ann Close, Nursing Director, The Dudley Group of Hospitals NHS Trust

Bridgit Dimond – MA, LLB, DSA, AHSM, Barrister-at-Law and Emeritus Professor at the University of Glamorgan

Derek Eaves, Clinical Governance Coordinator, The Dudley Group of Hospitals NHS Trust

Anne Flavell, Ward Manager, Trauma Orthopaedic Unit, The Dudley Group of Hospitals NHS Trust

Amanda Gethin, Ward Manager, The Dudley Group of Hospitals NHS Trust

Gill Henn. Tissue Viability Nurse Specialist, The Dudley Group of Hospitals NHS Trust

Briony Howells, Matron, Emergency Centre, The Dudley Group of Hospitals NHS Trust

Dr. Rebecca Jester, Associate Dean, School of Health University of Wolverhampton, Mary Seacole Building, City Campus Wolverhampton.

Dr. M.H Labib Consultant Pathologist, The Dudley Group of Hospitals NHS Trust

S.L. Labib, Sister in Critical Care, The Dudley Group of Hospitals NHS Trust

Linda M.Raybould, Lead Infection Control Nurse (Matron) The Dudley Group of Hospitals NHS Trust.

Jeanette Welsh, Practice Development Nurse, The Dudley Group of Hospitals NHS Trust

This book is dedicated

to the memory of Amanda Gethin,

who is sadly missed by

her many colleagues

The editors and publisher gratefully acknowledge the permission granted to reproduce the copyright material in this book. Every effort has been made to trace copyright holders and to obtain their permission for the use of copyright material. The publisher apologizes for any errors or omissions in this book and would be grateful if notified of any corrections that should be incorporated in future reprints or editions.

Introduction

Over the past ten years, the NHS has embarked on a journey of reform to ensure that the service provides a high standard of care; meets patients' needs and expectations; is provided in a safe, reassuring environment; and becomes more efficient and effective, providing value for money. As a result, the demands on nurses working in clinical practice have increased beyond the delivery of direct patient care.

This book has been written largely by staff working in a busy acute district general hospital, who understand what it is like to juggle all the priorities and demands made of them.

We have structured the book into four parts to help nurses manage patient care in the hospital from admission to discharge; make the patients' environment safe and welcoming; understand how they can use techniques to develop and improve the quality of care; and, finally, to consider what their roles and responsibilities are, what others expect from them (both inside and outside the hospital) and how they plan, develop and achieve their career goals.

It is intended that nurses can dip into and out of the chapters to help them address problems and concerns in a practical way as they arise. We have included a section entitled 'Remember what you can do' in each chapter, which summarises the key priorities.

We hope you will find this text helpful in your busy working lives providing clinical care for patients in hospital.

Ann Close and George Castledine

Section 1
The patient's perspective

The patient's perspective

Coming into hospital can be a frightening experience for any patient and their family. Hospitals are alien places for most people with their own written and unwritten rules. Instead of being in their home or workplace with familiar faces around them and well practised routines, they find that everyone is a stranger. They don't know what is expected of them, what they are 'allowed' to do, or what they should have brought with them. In addition to this, patients are worried about their illness or condition and the prospect of the treatment and nursing care they will receive.

The environment can have a significant effect on people — the unique smells, the different noises, the need to share rooms and facilities, the general hustle and bustle and the unfamiliar language used by many of the staff. Being asked to remove day clothing and wear nightwear often results in a feeling of loss of identity and loss of control over what is happening to them. This may lead to disorientation or confusion particularly in older people. Patients meet a lot of different staff during the course of their hospital stay and frequently find different titles and uniforms confusing.

Patients may also feel lonely and isolated from family and friends at a time when they need them the most. They may find there is a lot of waiting and sitting around but they haven't the energy, motivation or concentration to read or do other activities and instead they may sit and worry.

Nurses should remember how such experiences can affect a patient's behaviour. Family members are frequently concerned and anxious and naturally they focus on their relative as the priority. This can affect their behaviour too. Effective communication is therefore essential to provide patients and family members not only with information about what is happening, but also provide the opportunity to discuss and ask questions and, if necessary, have it repeated. It will help if you try to put yourself in the patient's and relatives' place.

This section is intended to help you manage patient care in the hospital environment from admission to discharge. *Chapter 1 Admission and discharge* looks at the route of admission, the initial assessment, the importance of communication and the key issues you will need to consider in the discharge process. *Chapter 2 Managing patient care* covers the role of the nurse in ensuring that the management of the patient's nursing care meets the highest standard available and links with the overall plan of care for the patient. It also identifies the steps you should take in assessing, planning, implementing, and evaluating care. *Chapter 3* provides guidance on documentation and standards for documenting care and suggests how handover reports should be conducted. *Chapter 4 Clinical rounds* describes two types of rounds – nurse management rounds and patient comfort rounds aimed at bringing back the patient focus to care. Both of these have their roots in the past but have been revised to reflect nursing and health care today.

Chapter 5 Customer care will help you in developing effective professional relationships with patients, relatives and others and responding to queries and complaints including the help that PALS (Patient Advice and Liaison Service) can offer. The principles put forward in *Chapter 6 Managing emergencies* will help you cope more effectively with some of the emergency situations that will occur during the course of your daily work. *Chapter 7 Wound care* describes one of the major nursing challenges of wound management and describes stages of wound healing, wound assessment and prevention. *Chapter 8 Interpretation of lab results* describes the commonest laboratory tests used and the causes of abnormal results that you will be likely to come across. *Chapter 9 Medicines management* looks at your role in the safe storage of medicines, good practice in administration and factors which contribute to errors and the action that you can take to minimise risks. *Chapter 10 Spiritual aspects of hospital nursing* aims to help you understand spirituality and how you might help patients with theirs. It also suggests pointers to assessing patients' and your own spirituality and how you and your colleagues can develop more spiritual awareness in your workplace. Finally, the chapter looks at loss, grief and bereavement in hospital, care of the dying patient and breaking bad news.

Chapter 1

Admission and discharge

Jo Parker

A stay in hospital can be a distressing time for individuals and their families and friends. Effective admission and discharge practices, including effective co-ordination with the agencies that provide care after discharge are important in reducing the stress of a hospital stay for all concerned and enhancing continuity of care and rehabilitation. This chapter looks at the route of admission, the initial assessment on admission, the importance of communication and the key issues to consider in the discharge process.

Admission

Patients may be admitted to hospital in a number of ways:

- **Routine admission.** The patient's admission is planned for, either for tests, surgery or other treatment.
- **Emergency admission.**
- **Direct GP referral.** The patient sees their general practitioner who refers to the hospital and the patient is admitted.
- **Domiciliary visit** where a consultant visits the patients at home and arranges admission.
- Patient is admitted from the **out-patient clinic**.
- **Patient self refers** through the emergency department and is admitted.

Initial assessment

You should make an initial assessment of the patient by simple observation. Check the patient's:

- breathing rate and pattern
- temperature
- blood pressure

- oxygen saturation levels
- appearance for pallor and whether they appear to be in pain.

Assess the risk of them developing a pressure sore and remember to take into account the individual's nutritional status. You should be aware of and use any tools approved by your organization. The single assessment process being implemented as one of the targets for the National Service Framework (NSF) Older People (DoH, 2001) will help in this process. Your assessment should be documented clearly and immediate preventative measures should be taken. A more detailed assessment and care plan can be carried out at a later stage (Chapter 2).

Important patient information

On admission remember things that will be important to your patients:

- vicinity of toilets/washing facilities.
- ward visiting hours.
- how to work the nurse call system.
- information on condition and tests.
- opportunity to express fears and or anxieties.
- opportunity to ask questions. They probably want to know:
  - ❖ what is wrong with them?
  - ❖ how long they will be in hospital?
  - ❖ what will happen to them?

Record keeping

Keep all records in one place to avoid unnecessary duplication and subsequent delays. Make sure you keep these confidential.

Communication with patients and carers

Effective communication is important with patients and carers at all times during the hospital stay but particularly on admission and discharge. You should:

- use plain English with no technical jargon
- seek permission from the patient to share information with their relatives

or carers.

- ensure that each patient and carer understand the procedures that they are having, and the reasons why
- give information sheets and ensure there is ample time for patients and carers to read them. Make time to go back and answer any questions. Remember these are not a substitute for information you can give them
- ensure that your admission assessment is thorough, ie. does it have a knock-on effect on anything else. For instance, is the patient looking after someone at home? Do they have pets? Is their anything worrying them which is not directly related to their admission that could affect their recovery?

Interpreters

Do not assume that if your patient cannot speak English that they will be happy for a member of their family to interpret for them. You cannot always rely on the accuracy of information provided. Check to see if there are approved interpreters used by your organisation and when appropriate contact them. Individual hospitals will have procedures for contacting interpreters.

Communication aids

There should be a variety of communication aids to assist patients, such as:

- large print
- braille
- British sign language
- audio Tapes
- cd roms
- appropriate ethnic minority languages.
- pictures.

Discharge

It is increasingly evident that effective hospital discharges can be best achieved when there is good joint working between staff groups and agencies including the NHS, local authorities, housing organizations, primary care and the independent and voluntary sectors.

The main problems arising from discharges have been identified in *Discharge from Hospital, pathways processes and practices* (DoH, 2003) and are because they:

- **occur too soon** — there may be pressure on acute beds but home, intermediate care services or rehabilitation are not available immediately
- **are delayed** — these problems often arise because of internal hospital factors such as waiting for tests and results, or delays in referring for home assessments or in getting medications. Patients and their families are also involved in the process and their taking time to decide on their future care can add to delays
- **are poorly managed from the patient and carer perspective** — if no account is taken of the patient's wishes and circumstances or if patients have not been kept informed of plans.
- **are to unsafe environments** — for example where the patient is unable to manage.

Delayed discharges

This occurs often when the continuing care required by frail, vulnerable, older people is uncertain and they remain in an acute hospital ward until decisions are made about their future. However an acute hospital ward is not a good place for them to remain once their acute episode of illness is over and measures are being put in place to reduce delays in discharge.

You are likely to hear the term 'whole system approach' to managing care. This aims to place the patient at the centre of service provision and respond to their needs. It aims to avoid unnecessary hospital admission, to promote good clinical outcomes and effective discharge planning with organizations working proactively, separately and together, to review and improve performance and find solutions.

The Government has also introduced a reimbursement scheme (Community Care Act 2003). The aim of which is to:

- improve local authority assessment and service provision through financial incentives
- encourage transfer to community settings
- encourage collaboration on equipment and intermediate care.

NHS bodies now have a new duty of care to notify social services of patients who have the likely need for services and a proposed discharge date. There are defined timescales for social services to complete assessments and provide services. Local authorities will have to reimburse acute trusts if discharge plans are not complete or if social care services are not available.

Important factors in discharge planning

- Involvement of patients and their families and carers is important. Remember they are individuals who have a good understanding of their own needs and the ability to influence their discharge process.
- Planning for hospital discharge is part of an ongoing process and should occur at the earliest possible opportunity and, if possible, prior to admission. Pre-admission assessment can help patients and their families understand how they can help themselves contacting the appropriate agencies early can avoid many problems. Advising relatives of an approximate length of stay and implementing the single assessment process will also help this (DoH 2001).
- On admission it is important to identify those patients who have additional health, social or housing needs and will need extra support.
- A patient's discharge should be the responsibility of one person, such as the key worker, named nurse, the primary nurse, the discharge co-ordinator.This will ensure all stages of the process are carried out correctly and reduce problems caused by poor communication or handover.
- The discharge should follow a clear, well defined pathway and adhere to the policy and procedures of the organization and local health economy which should involve the multidisciplinary team and all relevant agencies.
- An understanding is needed of transitional and intermediate care, and of rehabilitation services.
- Communication is easier where common records are in use.

Current level of support

In planning the patients discharge you need to consider:

- is your patient currently receiving support, eg. from social services?
- does the patient perceive the service input as adequate?
- does the carer perceive the service as adequate?
- check the patient's family support network.
- is the reason for admission going to affect the patient's activities of daily living on a short-term basis, not at all, or on a long-term basis?

These will help you determine whether referral to other agencies is necessary. You will also need to check:

- transport home. This should be well organized and timely and may be provided by:
  - ❖ family members collecting the patient
  - ❖ hospital taxi
  - ❖ ambulance. Get a booking reference number when booking and ensure that everything is ready to reduce unnecessary waiting times of ambulance crews.

Referring to agencies

The referrals you make will vary depending on the needs of the patients and what is available in your area. You should be aware of your responsibilities for making referrals.

Occupational therapist

If appropriate find out as soon as possible after the patient's admission what the system is for referral.

- Ensure that details in the referral are completed fully to avoid unnecessary delays.
- Have realistic outcomes. The occupational therapist will assess the individual's activities of daily living and determine whether the patient will be able to cope at home.
- The occupational therapist will be able to recommend and order equipment that will make the individual's life easier, ie. bath boards and commodes. Delivery of equipment should be in advance wherever possible.
- You will need to assess whether the family requires any training on the use of equipment, eg. hoists, beds, grab rails and arrange this with the occupational therapist.
- If there is a need for adaptations to the individual's home you will need to know the local arrangements for disabled facilites grants. The funding varies across the country and with the ownership of the property. Where work on adaptations takes longer than planned you may need to make arrangements for alternative care.

Community nurses

Each hospital has its own method of referring to the community nursing service. Have a working knowledge of your own procedure. Check if this is done by:

- telephone
- letter
- fax (patient identification labels do not fax well).This method is useful in avoiding delays.
- email
- liaison nurse who visits the ward and collects referrals on a daily basis
- when completing referral forms be thorough and specify precisely what is required
- always be conscious of the Data Protection Act (1998)
- be specific about when you want the service to start and how often visits are required
- check whether any pieces of equipment are required, eg. suture removal equipment
- if specific dressings are needed make sure you know your hospital's policy on what they will supply. A list should be available from the pharmacy. Find out where the patient can get anything not on the list.

Referral to social services

Each hospital will have an agreed procedure for referral to social services. You should have a good working knowledge of this so that you can make referrals at the earliest opportunity. You should also be aware of:

- the information social workers require and if specific forms need to be completed
- whether assessment by medical or therapy colleagues needs to be complete before referral
- what the agreed response times by social services are.

Other referrals

You may need to make referrals to other healthcare professionals such as dieticians, speech and language therapists or chiropodists and you should be aware of your hospital's procedures for doing this.

Ordering of tablets to take home (TTOs)

Check your trust's policy.

- Do all of the patient's own drugs need to be supplied again, or just the ones newly prescribed? If you are supplying the patient's tablets as TTOs make that the patient understands that they are instead of the ones they brought into hospital. If there has been any change in the way the tablets are to be taken, make sure that the patient is clear about this.
- Can they be ordered in advance to avoid delays on the day of discharge?
- The patient's general practitioner needs up-to-date information so that their revised plan of care can continue at home. Discharge letters need to be sent to the patient's GP as soon as possible.

Communication on discharge

Patients and their carers need information verbally and in writing when they leave hospital about:

- their condition, care and treatment
- medication
- care arrangements, ie. transitional and intermediate
- transport arrangements
- follow-up arrangements. How to access signers and interpreters if appropriate
- benefits available and any costs for care they are likely to face
- activities, driving, return to work, shopping, housework etc and when they can start these
- equipment or aids, how to use them and what to do if they don't work or are no longer needed
- information about support already arranged, eg. community nursing
- what to do if there are problems. Contact numbers should be given
- other sources of help and support such as self-help groups, PALS and advocacy support
- how to access the hospital complaints procedure.

Carers will also need information about:

- Support networks for them.
- What is expected of them as carers and how to undertake specific aspects of care. Demonstrate the use of equipment and ensure the carer is competent and confident to use it.

- Contact numbers for help and support
- Carers UK can provide help and information for carers on their website www.carersonline.co.uk . Advice line 08088087777
- The Princess Royal Trust can also provide information on the local services to support carers. Contact via the above website or by telephone 0207480 7788

Special circumstances

Homeless people

- Homeless people should be identified on admission and their pending discharge notified to the relevant primary healthcare services and to the homeless service providers.
- People aged sixty-five and under should be referred to the local homeless unit.
- People aged sixty-five and over to social services.

Self-discharge

- Check your local policy.
- Is your patient of sound mind to fully understand the implications of self-discharge?
- What can you do to ensure the patient's safety?

Remember what you can do

- Involve patients families and carers in admission and discharge.
- Make sure patients and their carers are provided with information that they can understand and refer to.
- Be aware of your local discharge policy and the need to keep up to date with changes in it.
- Be aware of your responsibilities in the discharge process.
- Keep up to date with the options available to patients on discharge — transitional care, intermediate care, rehabilitation etc.

- Have a working knowledge of how colleagues in the multidisciplinary team and other agencies contribute to a successful patients discharge.
- Remember the importance of communication in ensuring successful discharge.

References

Department of Health (2001) *The national service framework for older people*. DoH, London

Department of Health (2003) *Discharge from Hospital — pathway process and practice*. DoH, London

The Community Care (delayed discharges) Act. April 2003

The Data Protection Act 1998

Additional reading

Atwal A (2002) Nurses perceptions of discharge planning in acute health care: a case study in one British Teaching Hospital. *J Adv Nurs* **39**(5): 450–8

Carers England (2002) Hospital discharge practice briefing. Carers UK, London

DoH (2001) Continuing Care: NHS and local councils responsibilities (HSC2001/015: LAC(2001)18) DoH, London

Roberts K (2002) Exploring participation: older people on discharge from hospital. *J Adv Nurs* **40**(4): 413–20

Rudd C, Smith J (2002) Discharge Planning. Nurs Standard **17**(5): 33–7

Sutcliffe A, Potter A (2002) Multidisciplinary pre-admission clinics for orthopaedic patients. *Nurs Standard* **16**(21): 39–42

Werrett J, Carnwell R (2001) The primary and secondary care interface: the educational needs of nursing staff for the provision of seamless care. *J Adv Nurs* **34**(51): 629–38

Useful websites

www.carersonline.org   Carers UK
www dh.gov.nhs.uk   Department of Health

Chapter 2

Managing patient care

George Castledine

Nursing, like medicine and the other healthcare professions, is evolving and adapting to meet the demands of healthcare in society today. Although hospitals are changing, they still provide a vital role in the health care of any society. Hospitals are specialised places in which to recover from both illness and surgery and patients need careful and considerate management. It is nursing's responsibility and duty to ensure that a patient's nursing care management meets the highest standards available and that it links in with the overall plan of care for the patient. Collaboration and inter-professional team working are key words for all healthcare professionals.

This chapter describes how the nursing process should be used in the management and delivery of care. It includes the steps in the process and the key points to success. It also suggests assessment tools to use and emphasises the importance of psychosocial and mental health assessment in addition to physical assessment.

The nursing process

Using the nursing process to create a plan of care or patient care pathway provides a structure for nursing practice management and is the basis on which all nursing care is implemented. The nursing process is a dynamic system that can be used to explore the more intricate aspects of individual patients, their holistic needs and the unique outcomes of their health care. It should be put to use continuously during the implementation of nursing care in every clinical setting. When the nursing process became accepted in British nursing it was generally seen as a four-step process of assessment, planning, implementation and evaluation. Nowadays it is better to divide the assessment stage into two:

- **Gathering data** – this involves the nurse collecting data from a variety of sources, eg. interviewing the patient and their relatives, examining the patients and speaking to community, health and social care workers.

- **Problem identification** — this involves the nurse analysing all the available information and then deciding what are the patient's priorities and needs. This is sometimes referred to as making the nursing diagnosis. It is a critical stage because it highlights the differences between the nurse's perception and the patient's own perception of their problems and needs..

It is important to consider the patient as the central figure in any plan of care or pathway. The model shown in *Figure 2.1* illustrates that the nursing process is an interactive and dynamic action which is constantly changing, overlapping and repeating itself, depending on the individual patient's health, environment and management needs.

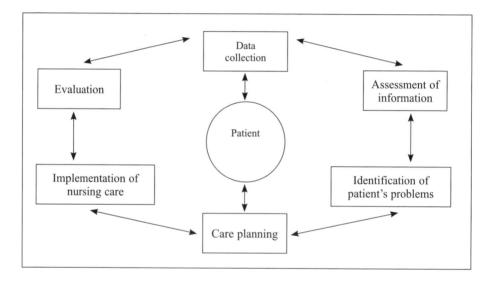

Figure 2.1: The nursing process

Steps of the nursing process

The following is a brief description of what you do at each stage.

1. Assessment

Gathering data:

- Carry out interviews of the patient, their relatives, friends and other workers who know the patient.
- Look for evidence of difficulty in function and the need for nursing care.
- Perform a physical assessment using all your senses and a systematic approach to collect information about your patient's health.
- Remember to look for psychosocial factors and spiritual needs.
- Emphasise the patient's strengths and involve them as much as possible.

Problem identification (nursing diagnosis)

- Analyse the collected information.
- Identify:
  - actual and potential problems
  - what the patient can and cannot do for themselves
  - the patient's priorities
  - the patient's risk of injury
  - the potential for self-care following discharge
  - patient and family education needs
  - any living will or statements relating to treatment and resuscitation.

Planning

Decide on:

- which core care plans and pathways should be used?
- which special patient monitoring charts are needed, eg. diabetic, fluid balance, pain and vital signs?
- how the patient's priorities are going to be met
- what the nurse should focus on when using the multidisciplinary care plans.
- what the patient can do for themselves?

- Develop expected outcomes or results for the patient.
- Determine what nursing care will be most appropriate for the patient.
- Think about the evidence which supports nursing actions and interventions.
- Remember the importance of documenting nursing care plans.

Implementation

This step in the process is all about putting the plans of nursing care into action. It involves regularly reviewing each day and in some cases, each shift, the plans of care for the patient.

There is a need to check that the patient is involved and aware of what is happening. The nurse needs to thinks carefully about:

- the best method of delivering the care, ie. patient assignment, team nursing or task allocation?
- when and how it is appropriate to delegate?
- how to monitor the patient's responses to interventions
- when and how to document and record the patient's responses and progress
- when to carry out and link together the variety of nursing actions to achieve holistic care
- how to co-ordinate and communicate with the rest of the healthcare team.

Evaluation

The nursing care should be evaluated regularly. In many cases this means delivering a good verbal report at shift handover and writing up the patient's progress in the nursing notes.

The nurse needs to question:

- how far the patient has met their expected outcomes
- in what ways things could be improved
- how is the physical and psychological care related to each other
- whether the care is becoming too fragmented and not dealing directly with the patients needs
- whether the patient is ready to manage their own care
- the effect of patient education and teaching
- plans for the patient's discharge or transfer?
- critically about what is happening to the patient at all times.

Evaluation is closely linked to planning and the need to review and audit nursing's contribution to patient care.

Critical thinking

Central to carrying out the nursing process is the knowledge base of the nurse and their ability to think critically. Thinking critically involves handling information in an analytical way to determine the patient's priorities and what the broad categories into which they fit, eg. daily living activities, functional problems, psychological problems, social problems, spiritual concerns.

Nursing assessment – key points to success

There are two types of data: objective and subjective.

Objective data: is obtained through observation and is verifiable, eg. oedema of the ankles and dry inelastic skin.

Subjective date: cannot be verified by anyone other than the patient, eg.pain and discomfort.

Nursing assessment involves:

a) interviewing the patient or their relatives and taking a health history including key nursing care issues
b) performing a physical assessment looking for key nursing care issues
c) teaching the patient about their body and nursing care needs when carrying out reassessments or more specialist physical and psychosocial techniques.

a) Interviewing the patient

Key sections of this interview should focus on:

■ Biographic data such as name, address, telephone number, birth date, age, marital status, religion and nationality, who the person lives with and the name and telephone number of a person to contact in the case of an emergency.
■ The patient's chief medical complaints, their understanding of it and their related nursing needs.
■ The patient's functional nursing needs for maintaining their activities of daily living.

■ Psychosocial and spiritual history, focusing on how the patient feels about themselves, their relationships with others, occupation, cultural background, handicaps and learning difficulties, beliefs and attitudes, especially any opinions and wishes related to resuscitation, nursing care and healthcare treatments.

b) Performing a nursing physical assessment

This involves the nurse examining the patient from two perspectives. Firstly to review the medical facts and secondly and, most importantly, to find out the patient's nursing needs.

It involves the nurse using her senses (ie. touch smell, sight and hearing) and approaching the patient in the following systematic way.

Firstly taking a step back and carefully performing an observational overview or general survey of the patient:

- reviewing the patient's general appearance
- mobility, movement and posture
- general skin condition
- height, weight and body mass.

NB: a patient's behaviours and appearance can offer subtle clues about their health and nursing needs.

Secondly, obtain baseline observations about the patient's temperature, pulse, respiration and blood pressure. In some cases it may also be essential to perform specialist observations such as neurological state in head injury patients (*Chapter 6*).

Thirdly, follow a simple systematic pattern such as, starting with the patient's hands and arms, moving to their head and covering their body and systems as you proceed from head to toe and back to the patient's hands (*Fig 2.2*).

Some experienced nurses may use the four techniques of inspection, palpation, percussion and auscultation. The most important techniques, however, are observation, inspection and handling the patient. This is enhanced if the patient is encouraged to change position so that the nurse gets a good sight of any relevant nursing needs and potential problems such as pressure areas on buttocks and problems in the patient's groins.

A common mistake by nurses when carrying out physical assessment is that they fail to check the inside of the patient's mouth, their breasts, buttocks, groins and feet, including toes and nails.

As the nurse assesses each part of the patient's body it is important therefore to check for colour, size, location, movement, texture, symmetry, odour and sounds.

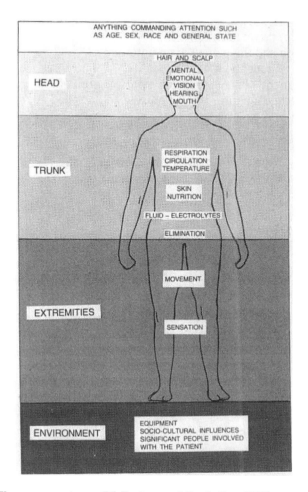

Figure 2.2: The assessment man (McFarlane and Castledine, 1982)

c) Reassessing and performing more in depth specialist nursing assessment

After the initial nursing assessment of a patient, it is important to continue to monitor the patient and reassess their condition.

Interviewing tips

■ Establish a rapport with the patient – explain the purpose of your questions and who you are.

- Choose a quiet private setting.
- Make sure you and the patient are comfortable.
- Reassure the patient about confidentiality.
- Assess the patient's language and general background; take into consideration age, culture, ability to listen and respond appropriately.
- Speak slowly and clearly.
- Listen carefully to answers.
- Make notes.
- Watch for non-verbal cues and that the patient is comfortable.
- Be aware of how you present yourself and ask questions.

Open-ended questions

- Encourage the patient to express feelings opinions and ideas.
- Use key words such as:
  - what
  - how
  - why
  - describe
  - where.

Closed questions

- These are used for quick short replies, eg:
  - do you?
  - is this?
  - are you?
  - did that?
  - has?

Other techniques

Use:

- **silence** to encourage the patient to talk and reflect on your questions
- **facilitation** to encourage story and history telling
- **confirmation** to check things
- **reflection** — to help the patient think things over

- **clarification** to confirm you have understood
- **summarising** — to sum up at the end what you have found out.

Encouraging patients to talk

Ask:

- is there something on your mind?
- what is it you would like to say?
- is there anything you would like to share with me?
- would you like to talk about it?

Or encourage with:

- I am here to listen, please go on.

Physical indicators of acute or chronic pain

- Noisy breathing.
- Negative vocalisation.
- Sad facial expression.
- Frowning.
- Tense body language.
- Fidgeting.

It is important to observe the patient carefully for these signs of pain. Remember that the patient's pain is what they say it is. A pain scale can be a very useful tool to determine how severe the patient's pain is. Also encourage the patient to express what word best describes the type of pain in simple terms.

No pain   1   2   3   4   5   6   7   8   9   10   Unbearable

Examples of words which best describe pain: dull ache, burning, pinching, throbbing, stabbing.

Psychosocial history

Ask about:

- previous history of mental health and coping in emotional crises
- any recent changes in personality or behaviour
- type and source of emotional support
- ability to exercise
- financial situation
- anything else concerning them.

Mental health assessment

Some key areas to assess:

- patient's physical appearance
- how they respond to the interview
- how well they cooperate
- the degree of agitation and activity
- swings and changes in mood
- thought processes
- level of alertness and orientation
- any suicidal or psychotic trends
- their insight and judgement.

The anxious patient

'Fear' is a key element of the anxious person. It may be accompanied by physical signs which affect the autonomic nervous system.

Two types of anxiety — normal and pathological may present. It is important to assess if the patient has any life-threatening conditions or reasons for being anxious.

- Assess:
  - patient's presenting symptoms
  - any medical illnesses
  - medication history
  - drug or alcohol misuse

- any history of mental illness
- patient's vital signs.
- Nurse the patient in a safe and quiet environment.
- Observe and monitor carefully.
- Encourage the patient to express and verbalise their concerns.

The depressed patient

Depression is a dispirited or dejected mood with loss of interest and pleasure. People with depression usually complain of helplessness, hopelessness, feeling worthless, 'down in the dumps' and much worse than when they were sad in the past.

- Assess:
  - what the patient says about themselves and their ability to cope
  - sleep patterns
  - gastrointestinal functioning
  - any recent causes such as shock, survival guilt, bereavement or loss
  - suicide tendencies or self-harm potential
  - the patient's appearance
  - general behaviour such as agitation, social withdrawal and isolation
  - any psychotic symptoms
  - any pain.

Geriatric depression scale (GDS)

This can be used to identify depression in the elderly population such as:

- pessimistic feelings
- concerns with physical health
- differences in mood
- lack of motivation
- loss of self-esteem
- cognitive difficulties
- feelings of discrimination
- loss of dignity.

	Geriatric depression scale		
1	Are you basically satisfied with your life?	Yes	No
2	Have you dropped many of your activities and interests?	Yes	No
3	Do you feel that your life is empty?	Yes	No
4	Do you often get bored?	Yes	No
5	Are you hopeful about the future?	Yes	No
6	Are you bothered about thoughts you can't get out of your head?	Yes	No
7	Are you in good spirits most of the time?	Yes	No
8	Are you afraid that something bad is going to happen to you?	Yes	No
9	Do you feel happy most of the time?	Yes	No
10	Do you often feel helpless?	Yes	No
11	Do you often get restless and fidgety?	Yes	No
12	Do you prefer to stay at home, rather than going out and doing new things?	Yes	No
13	Do you frequently worry about the future?	Yes	No
14	Do you feel you have more problems with memory loss than most?	Yes	No
15	Do you think it is wonderful to be alive now?	Yes	No
16	Do you often feel down-hearted and blue?	Yes	No
17	Do you often feel pretty worthles the way you are now?	Yes	No
18	Do you worry a lot about the past?	Yes	No
19	Do you find life very exciting?	Yes	No
20	Is it hard for you to get started on new projects	Yes	No
21	Do you feel full of energy?	Yes	No
22	Do you feel that your situation is hopeless	Yes	No
23	Do you think that most people are better off than you are?	Yes	No
24	Do you frequently get upset over little things?	Yes	No
25	Do you frequently feel like crying	Yes	No
26	Do you have trouble concentrating	Yes	No
27	Do you enjoy getting up in the morning?	Yes	No
28	Do you prefer to avoid social gatherings?	Yes	No
29	Is it easy for you to make decisions	Yes	No
30	Is your mind as clear as it used to be?	Yes	No
	Number of depressive answers (shaded boxes)		

Figure 2.2: Geriatric depression scale (Brink *et al*, 1982 and Yesavage *et al*, 1983)

First published in Brink TL, Yesavage JA, Lum O, Heersema P, Adley MB, Rose TL (1982) Screening tests for geriatric depression. *Clin Gerontol* 1: 37-44, reproduced by permission of Cambridge University Press

The violent and aggressive patient

Causes of violent and aggressive behaviour are complex. They may be due to psychiatric reasons, medical factors, family history, social history and past history of hostility in the face of stressful events.

The single best predictor of future violence is past violence. If a patient has an established history of violent or aggressive conduct, proceed with extreme care.

- Assess:
    - what and how the person says something – often they will express rage and anger about certain subjects, eg. a person or an establishment
    - is the patient verbally threatening?
    - is the situation getting worse?
    - is the patient on drugs or abusing alcohol?
    - is the patient listening?
    - what is the source of the patient's distress?
- Consider your situation and the need for a show of force (ie. call in the security team.
- Assess the patient and observe for any type of weapon or object that could be used as such.
- Approach the patient slowly in a relaxed manner with your hands visible.
- Don't make quick or hurried movements.
- Always remain three to six feet away from the patient.
- Stand sideways, ready to pivot away or dodge.
- Don't turn your back on the patient or get trapped away from the exit of a room.
- If the patient is amenable to verbal redirection – invite them to sit down and talk
- Always speak slowly, calmly and firmly.

The psychotic patient

Psychosis is a term used in psychiatry to describe a specific type of psychotic disorder. The patient who is suffering psychosis is unable to think clearly, respond emotionally, communicate reasonably, perceive and interpret reality or behave appropriately.

Psychosis may be associated with severe medical conditions and may result in aggression and unsociable behaviour.

- Assess
  - appearance and general hygiene
  - signs of agitation, severe restlessness, pacing, tremors and abnormal movements
  - quality of speech
  - rapidly changing behaviour such as aggressive, depressed or euphoric displays
  - changing thought processes, eg. flight of ideas
  - perceptions, hallucinations (visual, auditory, tactile or olfactory).
  - paranoid thinking, delusions of grandiosity or persecution and obsessions
  - changes to insight and judgement.

The confused patient

Acute confusion is very common in hospital patients. In general it is a state of being bewildered with what is going on around them and mistaking one person or a thing for another. All patients may be forgiven for being a little disorientated when they are hospitalised.

Severe cases of acute confusion can be caused by the presence of an acute medical problem such as:

- hypoglycaemia
- fever
- alcohol withdrawal
- drug reaction or intoxication
- head injury
- recent surgery.

Acute confusion is sometimes referred to as delirium. Its main symptoms to look out for are:

- agitation and restlessness
- hallucinations and delusions
- disorientation
- mood changes
- occasional aggression.

Acute confusion is very common in elderly patients and is characterised by a rapid onset and a fluctuating course, with symptoms that worsen at night time.

Assessing confusion by various means is possible, but nurses should not overlook the importance of not overlooking the cognitive function of a patient.

A simple test for confusion is the following abbreviated mental test score developed by Gaind (1981).

(Score 1 for each correct answer. If patient scores below 7, then confusion or some form of mental dysfunction is a strong possibility.)
Ask patient:

1. Age.
2. Time (to nearest hour).
3. Address (for recall at the end of the test: this should be repeated by the patient to ensure that it has been heard correctly).
4. Year.
5. Name of hospital.
6. Recognition of two persons (eg. doctor/nurse).
7. Date of birth.
8. Year of First World War, or other significant event.
9. Name of present monarch or prime minister.
10. Count Backwards from 20–1 or recite backwards the months in a year.

The patient with dementia

Dementia is a term that describes a group of disorders that affects the brain and causes loss of memory, and an ability to think clearly, to understand words, recognise people, calculate, speak clearly and comprehensively and be orientated in time, place and person. It affects and impairs daily living activities and is progressive in nature.

Alzheimer's disease accounts for about 50 percent of dementia cases. Early stage signs are:

- loss of recent memory
- repetitive questions
- forgetting conversation
- impaired language
- disorientation
- personality changes.

Later signs are:
- severe memory impairment
- behavioural disturbances
- aggression
- wandering
- hyperactivity
- incontinence
- lack of inhibition
- delusions
- hallucinations.

Remember what you can do

- Ensure you are familiar with all steps of the nursing process.
- Find out what assessment tools are used in your organisation.
- Ask for help and advice from nurse specialists or senior colleagues in using the tools with which you are not familiar.
- Ask colleagues for critical and constructive feedback on your patient interviews, assessments, care plans and evaluation.
- Keep a reflective diary of problems you have encountered in managing patient care and discuss at your appraisal or in a clinical supervision session or discuss with your preceptor.
- Find out what training and updating sessions are available in your organisation.

References

Brink TL, Yesavage JA, Lum O Heersema P, Adey MB, Rose TL (1982) Screening tests for geriatric depression. *Clin Gerontol* **1**: 37–44

Gaind R (1981) Organic mental impairment in the elderly. *J R Coll Physicians Lond* **15**(3): 140–4

McFarlane J, Castledine G (1982) *A Guide to the Practice of Nursing Using the Nursing Process*. CV Mosby & Co, London

Yesavage JA, Brink TR, Rose TL, Lum O, Huang V, Adey MB, Leirer VO (1983) Development and validation of a geriatric depression screening scale; a preliminary report. *J Psychiatr Res* **17**(3): 37–49

Additional reading

Aird T, McIntosh M (2004) Nursing tools and strategies to assess cognition and confusion. *Br J Nurs* **13**(10): 621–6

Bird J (2003) Selection of pain measurement tools. *Nurs Standard* **18**(13): 33–9

Bourbonnais F *et al* (2004) Introduction of a pain and symptom assessment tool in the clinical setting. Lessons learned. *J Nurs Manag* **12**(3): 194–200

Briggs E (2003) The nursing management of pain in older people. *Nurs Standard* **17**(18): 47–55

Bryans M, Wilcock J (2001) Issues for nurses in dementia diagnosis and management. *Nurs Times* **97**(44): 30

Coll AM *et al* (2004) Post operative pain assessment tools in day surgery: literature review. *J Adv Nurs* **46**(2): 124–33

Davidhizar R *et al* (2004) A review of the literature on care of clients in pain who are culturally diverse. *Int Nurs Rev* **51**(1): 47–55

Manthorpe J *et al* (2003) Early recognition of dementia by nurses. *J Adv Nurs* **44**(2): 183–91

Murdock D (1997) The nursing process: a method of collecting evidence. *Nurs Standard* **11**(28): 40–1

Ruland C, Kresevic D, Lorensen M (1997) Including patient preferences in nurses assessment of older patients. *J Clin Nurs* **6**(6): 495–504

Taylor C (2002) Assessing patients' needs: does the same information guide expert and novice nurses. *Int Nurs Rev* **49**(1): 11–9

White S. (2004) Assessment of chronic neuropathic pain and the use of pain tools. *Br J Nurs* **13**(7): 372–8

Useful websites

www.rcn.org.uk	Royal College of nursing
www.nmc-uk.org	Nursing and Midwifery council
www.internurse.com	on-line archive of peer reviewed articles
www.nelh.nhs.uk	National Electronic Library for Health

Chapter 3

Documentation and handover reporting

George Castledine

As the healthcare delivery system in the UK continues to modernise and diversify, documentation of the actual care delivered to patients becomes more critical. The role of the hospital nurse today is changing and there are many new demands in addition to the traditional activities of the nurse. Some of these developments include performing more medical tasks and working more closely with other healthcare professionals in delivering integrated care pathways. This chapter provides guidance on documentation and standards for documenting care and suggests how handover reports should be conducted.

Patients in hospitals are much sicker and older than they used to be, which makes not only their medical problems more complex, but also their nursing problems. Often patients stay in hospital wards and clinical areas for just a few days or even for just a few hours. They are frequently transferred to different units during a single short stay and may move rapidly around a hospital, receiving a variety of treatments and health care. Establishing any form of meaningful therapeutic nurse-patient relationship is very difficult. The rapid turnover of patients has meant that many nurses have little time for adequate assessment and care planning.

Documentation is a vital link in presenting the true picture of a patient's stay in hospital and the outcomes of all nursing and medical interventions. Nursing documentation must reflect this by outlining clearly what happened to the patient on admission, their nursing assessment, individual needs, involvement in care, daily progress and their journey through the hospital system prior to transfer or discharge.

There are many different systems of documentation used within clinical facilities today. It is important to familiarise yourself with the particular system which is being used in your hospital.

Each hospital should have guidelines or standards relating to its needs. Remember documentation of patient care is a legal requirement in many countries and it needs to be legible and neat. Furthermore don't let your own standards be compromised and fall below what is generally expected.

The following information is aimed at trying to help you fulfil the fundamental requirements of nursing documentation.

Nursing documentation

Charts

The documentation which the nurse has to complete consists of filling in charts, either situated at the patient's bedside or contained in a special folder and kept at the nurses station. These charts are usually concerned with specific observations being carried out on the patient, such as, temperature, blood pressure recording, fluid balance, pain control, nutrition and neurological observations.

Care plans

Other documentation which the nurse is concerned with relates to the patient's care planning and drug administration. Again some of these may be kept near to the patient for easy access by the nurse or in special folders for use by all team members. Many wards and units are now using integrated care pathways (ICPs) and these plans are not only followed by all the hospital/ward teams but are also filled in by them and kept up to date with the patient's progress.

It is important that, whatever the documentation system, the nurse plays a vital role in keeping the process up to date and makes sure that there is a professional nursing contribution. During the charting or documentation process it is important that the nurse takes time to plan and organise what to enter into the record or on to the observation charts. Recording and writing up nursing observations should follow local and national guidelines such as those proposed by the Nursing and Midwifery Council (NMC). Descriptive and objective data should be recorded rather than data based on inferences, conclusions, assumptions and hearsay. The patient and their significant relatives and friends should be involved in documentation and there should be evidence of this in the records.

Documentation (charting) guidelines

Whenever a patient complains of a change in physical, mental or emotional status or is transferred to a new hospital ward, it is important to carry out a short five-minute assessment or reassessment of their health and nursing needs. The following will help you:

- Try and assess the patient not only quickly but also systematically.
- Careful explanation of what you are doing will help the patient to keep calm and promote co-operation.
- Think carefully about what you are observing and how you are going to organise and write up your observations.
- When recording the physical observations of the patient be accurate and concise.
- Organise your information so that it follows some type of logical progression, eg. head to toe observation.
- When you describe the patient's behaviour include only the facts and not personal opinions on why the person is behaving the way they are.
- Try and identify the patient's individual nursing problems and needs.
- Include patient responses to questions about their nursing care and health problems.
- Type or write neatly and legibly and in blue or black ink.
- Use good grammar, correct spelling, correct punctuation and proper terminology.
- Always record the date and time.
- When correcting or making a change to an entry in a computerised system enter the current time and date, identify yourself and note the reasons for the change.
- Never write up what you did not see, hear or personally experience with the patient.
- Never chart in advance of doing something: particularly when administering drugs, changing intravenous fluids or carrying out a nursing procedure.
- Try and chart as soon as possible after an observation or procedure.
- Use only those abbreviations accepted in your hospital.
- Patient care and the patient's condition should be regularly reassessed to form a diary of their progress through their hospital stay.
- Start recording information immediately so that eventual discharge of the patients and transfer home will not be delayed.
- Record the type of education and information the patient has received.
- At the end of the shift you should check through your patients' charts and be certain that all entries are complete and appropriately signed.

Handover reports

In recent years the time available for handover reports has decreased significantly. this is due to shorter overlap of shifts and nurses starting shifts at different times to meet patients' needs and their own family and personal commitments. Handover reports, therefore, have to be short and concise but at the same time pass on the essential information about the patient and their care. The following guidelines are intended to help you:

- Always refer to the written records and use them to check the accuracy of your statements and information.
- Identify the patient's main nursing problems and concerns.
- Stress how recent changes may have affected your care or will affect others in the future.
- Ensure that any bank, agency or new staff are briefed fully in the patient's problems and care needs.
- Do not become engaged in idle gossip and wander from the point of the report.
- Organise your thoughts and think carefully about how you will talk about the patients entrusted to you.
- Highlight any specific events which have happened to the patient during your shift.
- Present the patient's current condition and any relevant vital signs.
- Highlight any specific events that are planned during the next shift.
- Ensure you use the report to clarify any concerns or queries you might have about a patient's treatment or care.
- Behave professionally at all times and do not get dragged into unprofessional behaviour and gossip.

Some hospitals have introduced different ways of providing handover reports including taped handovers. These are particularly useful when there are several staff starting shifts at slightly difference times, as it prevents nurses from repeating the information several times to different nurses.

In the past, handovers were used to teach staff aspects of patient care. Time constraints have often seen this practice reduced but it may be possible to use the handover on one or two occasions a week to update or teach each other.

Conclusion

The art of documentation and charting develops with practice over time. It is essential that nurses are as accurate and rigorous about their nursing records as they can be. Any incompleteness and 'sloppy' practice may well be picked up by a jury as signs of poor professional conduct, bad record keeping and poor nursing care.

Remember what you can do

- Make sure you are aware of the standards and guidelines for documentation and record keeping for your organization.
- Read the NMC guidelines on records and record keeping.
- Find out if any audits are done on documentation in your area and, if not, suggest that you do one to find how well you meet the standards.
- Find out if there are any update sessions on documentation and record keeping in your organisation and, if not, ask for some to be arranged.
- Ask an honest colleague for a critical and constructive appraisal of your documentation and record keeping.

Additional reading

Hopkinson J (2002) The hidden benefit: the supportive function of the nursing handover for qualified nurses caring for dying people in hospital. *J Clin Nurs* **11**(2): 168–175

McKenna L (1997) Changing handover practices: one private hospitals experiences. *Int J Nurs Prac* **3**(2): 128–132

Modernisation Agency (2003) Essence of Care Benchmarks for record keeping. DoH, London.

Moloney R, Maggs C (1999) A systematic review of the relationships between written manual nursing care, record keeping and patient outcomes. *J Adv Nurs* 30: 51–7

Nursing and Midwifery Council (2005) Guidelines for Records and Record Keeping. NMC, London

Oili K, Eriksson K (2003) Evaluation of patients records as part of developing a nursing care classification. *J Clin Nurs* **12**(2): 198–205

Payne S, Hardy M (2000) Interaction between nurses during handover in elderly care. J Adv Nurs **32**(2): 277–285

Prouse M (1995) A study of the Use of Tape recorded handovers. *Nur s Times* **91**(49): 40–1

Roden C, Bell M (2002) Record keeping: developing good practice. *Nurs Standard* **17**(1): 40–2

Sexton A *et al* (2004) Nursing Handovers: do we really need them. *J Nurs Manag* **12**(1): 37–42

Taylor H (2003) An exploration of the factors that affect nurses' record keeping. *Br J Nurs* **12**(12): 751–8

Useful websites

www.nmc-uk.org	Nursing and Midwifery Council
www.modern.nhs.uk	Modernisation Agency
www.nelh.nhs.uk	National Electronic Library for Health

Chapter 4

Clinical rounds

Ann Close and George Castledine

Clinical rounds formed an important component of care prior to the late 1980s and were valued by patients, staff and visitors. They provide the opportunity to bring the patient focus back into nursing together with discipline and accountability. This chapter describes two types of rounds — nurse management rounds and patient comfort rounds. Both of these have their roots in the past but have been revised to reflect nursing and health care today.

Nurse management rounds

Nurses training and working in hospitals in the 1960s, '70s and early '80s may remember the ward sister or her deputy doing a round of the patients usually at the beginning of each shift and often at visiting times. In addition to a formal greeting, sister would ask how the patient was, whether they had slept, if they had any pain or discomfort, whether their bodily functions were in working order and other questions specifically relating to the patient's condition. In addition they would check fluid input and output, sputum, wounds, blood or drainage loss and vital signs appropriate to the patient.

Sister would also use the opportunity to give patients information about tests, procedures and other aspects of treatment they would be experiencing that day and remind them of doctors' rounds, visits by social workers and any specimens that were required.

This would take no more than a couple of minutes per patient and enabled sister to pick up any new information or condition change following the handover report and therefore served to give her an up-to-date overview of all patients on the ward on which to plan the day's work and be ready to act as patients' advocate and support during doctors' rounds. Sister would frequently take a student nurse with her and although she might do some teaching, most learning in this situation was by sister being a role model.

During the '70s and '80s a number of factors resulted in changes in the ward sister's authority and the demise of these rounds.

Patients' dissatisfaction

In the late 1980s patients began to complain that they did not know who was in charge of their care. Many patients gain considerable reassurance when they see the ward sister in charge of the ward. As a result the concept of primary nursing was promoted by the government in the *Strategy for Nursing* (DoH 1989). One of the ways of introducing this was the 'named nurse' and this approach was introduced in the *Patient's Charter* by the Government in October 1991 (DoH, 1991). This attempted to make it clear that the responsibility and accountability for care rested with the individual nurse. As a result, responsibility and accountability for care rested with the individually named nurse.

In essence, the named nurse is responsible for assessing, planning and evaluating care and coordinating the overall plan of care.

It can be argued that there are several potential benefits to the named nurse system, including an increased focus on the individual needs of patients who are clear as to who is responsible for their nursing care, improved job satisfaction for nurses and improved quality of care. However, the reality has been that there have been difficulties with implementation, particularly as a result of having insufficient staffing levels and skill mix to provide continuity of care and some patients may see their named nurse only once on admission.

Named nursing, therefore, with accountability firmly rooted in the individual nurse, further reduced the need for a coordinated team approach to care across the ward.

Healthcare professionals' dissatisfaction

Doctors experience frustration when doing their ward rounds as no one seems to take the overall responsibility for the patients on the ward. They are unable to find the right nurse who can provide up-to-date information on the patients' condition and progress and act as the patient's advocate. There is often no one to pass information on to or discuss the proposed treatment plan with. Communication is mostly through written notes in the patient's record resulting in some essential components being missed.

Other healthcare professionals experience similar situations when coming to treat patients. They have difficulty locating patients who have been referred to them and are passed from one nurse to the next with such comments as, 'Oh he's not my patient' or they find that the named nurse is on a break and no one has information about the patient in question.

Relatives' dissatisfaction

Relatives, too, experience difficulties. They may be unable to find out about the patient when they make telephone enquiries if the nurse looking after the patient isn't available or they don't know who to speak to when they have any concerns. This undermines their confidence in the care being provided.

Others' dissatisfaction

Other visitors, such as managers also experience similar problems when visiting wards to discuss patient care, complaints and other management issues. Nurses themselves are sometimes unaware of who is the most senior nurse in charge of the ward and the patients.

This situation results in a lack of leadership, poor organisation, priorities not being addressed and staff not always being managed in the best way. Introducing nursing management rounds can help improve the situation.

What are nursing management rounds?

The nurse in charge undertakes rounds of the patients – normally at the beginning of the shift – to get an overview of all their needs and the ability of staff to meet them. These are very much like the ward sisters rounds described at the beginning of the chapter.

The purpose of the nursing management rounds

The nurse in charge of the shift should see each patient for the following reasons.

To determine the condition of each patient:

- Patients in hospital today are frequently highly dependent with complex conditions, which can change rapidly. Although information will have been passed on at handover report, it is important that the nurse in   charge sees the patient to ensure that priorities are addressed and the most appropriate care given.

■ It provides opportunities to see if treatments and drug regimes are working; to check, for example, whether pain relief has been effective, the amount and type of wound drainage or to check post-operative progress. This information is not only important to plan nursing care but also to share with other healthcare professionals at ward rounds to determine whether a doctor or therapist should see a patient urgently and not wait until the regular round.

■ If patients are planned for discharge or transfer, seeing the patient will determine if they are fit or whether a change in plan is necessary.

■ If patients are going for tests, procedures or x rays, it will help determine what level of escort they require or if the mode of transfer has to change, say, from a wheelchair to a trolley.

To determine patients' concerns and anxieties:

■ Patients often worry about things that seem of minor importance to healthcare professionals and these are often sorted out easily if they are known about. They are also reluctant to ask questions and raise problems when they see nurses rushing about. However, if there is a regular time when the nurse in charge will be speaking to them they are more prepared to raise their concerns.

■ Minor irritations or dissatisfaction with aspects of care can escalate into complaints if they are not dealt with quickly. When one thing goes wrong for a patient they are often more alert to other things going wrong and will interpret events and behaviours in negative ways. If not addressed, complaints may result after discharge when there is no opportunity to put things right. In addition, it will take up considerable time for nursing staff to respond to the points raised in the formal complaint process.

To keep patients up to date with care treatment and progress:

■ Healthcare professionals often assume that patients know more about their care and treatment than they actually do. They forget that patients don't have the same grasp of health service jargon and often need information to be repeated to get a full picture of what is happening. Rounds by the nurse in charge can help to reinforce this information for the patient and, if any investigations or procedures are planned for the day, then these can be checked with the patient to ensure they are prepared. Similarly, reminders of visits by other specialist nurses, social workers and consultants can be made.

To determine if the care given meets the patients needs:

■ As part of the process of nursing there should be an evaluation of the patient's progress on an ongoing basis. The nurses should record the progress in the patient's record. Undertaking rounds provides an opportunity for a more senior and experienced nurse to check that care has been carried out to the agreed plan and documented accurately. This acts as an early warning system. If goals have not been met, or progress is slower than expected, questions can be asked as to why this may be the case and whether staff shortages, skills and knowledge deficit or workload issues are having an adverse effect. In such instances, changes to the allocation of workload or the redeployment of staff can be made to ensure priorities are addressed, or training and updating of practices may need to be planned. Alternatively, investigation may reveal that there is a deterioration in the patient's condition which may not have been detected previously. Appropriate action should be taken to ensure the patient's plan of care is reviewed or, if necessary, is seen by medical staff.

To ensure documentation and records are up to date and acted upon:

■ Nursing documentation should provide an accurate and comprehensive record of the patient's condition, the care required and delivered and progress made. This written documentation forms the basis of information communicated to members of the team to ensure continuity of care. To be effective, the records must be accurate, current, legible and complete. Documentation, records and charts can be checked during ward rounds so that they meet the standards set and any problems can be highlighted and omissions dealt with.

To ensure standards are being achieved

■ With the advent of evidence-based practice, clinical nurses are faced with new standards, guidelines, policies and procedures to incorporate into their day-to-day practice. Observation of practice, patient progress and outcomes and documentation and records during nurse management rounds will indicate whether nurses are working to the agreed standards and enable action to be taken if they are not.

To provide information

■ As patient's progress, they and their relatives often seek information about their life beyond hospital: what will happen to them, how can they expect to feel, what continuing care and treatment will be available. These can be identified during rounds and incorporated into the plan of care for the day. In addition, patients may have other health worries or financial and personal issues not relating to their current admission. Arrangements can be made for appropriate staff (such as from Cizens Advice Bureau) to visit with advice and information on, for example, health promotion or smoking cessation if nursing staff on the ward are not able to help.

Benefits of nursing management rounds

For patients families and carers

■ Rounds help them to identify who is in charge — this creates confidence and a feeling of security that there is one senior person with overall responsibility.
■ Rounds also help them to identify which nurses are caring for them during that shift.
■ There is increased accessibility to, and communication with, nurses in charge. Some patients and family members are reluctant to seek out those people they see in authority and therefore may not have their questions and worries addressed. Regular unsolicited contact should give them more opportunity and confidence to raise these.
■ Regular discussions may also help reduce complaints. If concerns and irritations are addressed, patient confidence and satisfaction will increase.
■ Sharing information and having discussions with patients and families can improve and speed up the discharge process.

The nursing team

- Nurse management rounds enable senior nurses to provide better supervision and support of their junior colleagues. They are more aware of all the patients' needs, the ability of the team to cope with these and are able to identify when staff might be struggling and ensure they get appropriate help.
- There should be improved communication with staff, not only about patients, but also about how well each member of the nursing team is performing. Senior nurses can give their staff immediate feedback and acknowledge the contribution they are making.
- Rounds provide opportunities for education and staff development and, as it is focused on the delivery of care, will be seen as relevant and important to staff which enhances their learning.
- These rounds will also provide staff with the opportunity to discuss problems with their senior colleagues and immediate ways of resolving them.
- They assist with the organisation of care and inform nurses about which patients they are caring for and the priorities during the shift.

Other healthcare professionals

- Nurse management rounds provide a focal point or person to liaise with – someone who is aware of all the patients' and relatives' issues and those raised by others in the healthcare team; someone who can support them when seeing patients and who can be relied on to coordinate the patient's care.

Principles for conducting nurse management rounds

- Normally, rounds will be undertaken at the beginning of the shift to highlight problems and where there is a need for more information. It will also provide the opportunity to check that documentation and charts are up to date from the previous shift. However this might not always be the case and each ward and department should decide which is best for the patients in that area.
- Rounds should be kept short. The aim is to be able to identify concerns that should be addressed during the shift by the team of nurses caring for

the patient or by members of the multidisciplinary team who can be asked to visit at a later stage.

■ It is important to remember confidentiality, privacy and dignity of patients. This can sometimes be difficult in ward and department environments and particularly sensitive discussions may need to be picked up later in a more private environment.

■ It is also important to remember control of infection principles and hand washing, in particular when moving between patients.

■ Common problems should be noted and discussed later with the team to identify education and training requirements.

■ The ward or department should develop a consistent approach to nursing management rounds, otherwise it may become confusing to patients, and staff if different approaches are used by different nurses when in charge.

Qualities required for undertaking nurse management rounds

Leadership

Nurse management rounds allow senior nurses to provide clinical and professional leadership to the more junior members of the team.

The ward or department sister/charge nurse, together with the staff, should set the values, direction and vision for patient care and the senior staff leading each shift are, responsible for instigating them in practice. This requires team spirit and team working which is achieved by ensuring each team member knows what is expected of them, what standards and values they are working to and the boundaries within which they should work. It also requires an understanding of members of the team, what drives them, what concerns them, what they enjoy and what they find difficult.

Communication

Effective communication skills are essential. During rounds staff must be able to talk to patients using jargon free language that they can easily understand. They must be able to pick up on non-verbal clues — which sometimes communicate a great deal about how a person is feeling — as well as listening to what the patient is saying without appearing hurried and distracted.

Senior staff must also be able to give clear instructions to more junior colleagues and be approachable so that staff feel able to seek clarification, guidance and receive constructive feedback.

Observation skills

Nurse management rounds demand effective observation skills to identify subtle, as well as more obvious, changes in patients' conditions. These skills are also necessary to check that documentation and record keeping is complete, accurate and up to date and that the patients' environment is clean and tidy.

Personal qualities

Shift leaders undertaking nurse management rounds should have considerable expertise in the care of patients in that area. Good organisational skills and a systematic approach to work will help them to undertake rounds efficiently and deal with actions arising from them. In addition, they should show commitment, flexibility, honesty and a willingness to train, guide and support team members.

Positive role model

All of the above will help the individual to become a positive role model. Junior staff will learn by observing and imitating senior colleagues during the course of their work and therefore senior staff can have a significant influence on the way junior staff develop.

Preparing and supporting staff to undertake nursing management rounds

Involving all staff in the team in deciding how nursing management rounds are implemented in a particular area is key to gaining their commitment. Ward managers and team leaders should work with the staff to plan how they will implement the rounds, who will undertake them, what preparation they require and how they will evaluate and monitor the process. They may also wish to consider what support mechanisms may be required.

It is essential that staff in charge of shifts understand the purpose and benefits of nursing management rounds as well as the principles involved. In addition they should be capable of doing them. Many of the qualities required can be developed through specific courses, individual training, guidance and coaching and by shadowing experienced individuals who are respected and positive role models.

Clinical supervision can be helpful in both supporting the individual and ensuring they reflect and learn from the experience. This would be helpful not only on a one-to-one basis but also through group supervision. Feedback may also be obtained from formal processes such as an appraisal or more informally from discussion with colleagues and patients.

Evaluating the benefits of nursing management rounds can be done through feedback from patients, their relatives, visitors, other healthcare professionals and staff undertaking the rounds. This can be through surveys, interviews, discussions, comments and suggestions and audit of records and documentation.

Patient comfort rounds

Patient comfort rounds (Castledine, 2002) are a new idea to help improve individual patient care on a ward or busy nursing unit. In the past, nurses used to carry out 'back rounds' which were associated with the prevention of bed sores. These would be performed regularly throughout the day and night on all patients who were restricted to their beds or chairs.

The rounds involved thoroughly washing the back, rubbing fairly vigorously and applying powder or a selection of solutions or creams such as silicone preparations. The practice died out in the majority of UK hospitals when it was found that two-hourly turning of the bedbound patients was more appropriate and nurse allocation systems were introduced.

Unfortunately, for various reasons — some associated with staffing shortages and increases in patient dependency and workloads — there is now a need to encourage closer monitoring of patient's individual nursing care.

The rounds are carried out two-hourly usually during the afternoon and evening following intensive nursing care in the morning when patients have been allocated to appropriate nurses. The aim is not to replace patient allocation but to supplement it by ensuring that nurses regularly review patients and tend to their basic needs. Whereas in the past the emphasis was on pressure sore prevention, today this is combined with a whole variety of holistic nursing functions (*see below*).

Content of patient comfort rounds

- Discussion with the patient and their relatives about the nursing interventions, plans and progress the patient is making.
- Attention to daily living activities and bodily functions such as hand hygiene, toileting and mouth care.
- Updating bedside charting and nursing observations and documentation.
- Adjustments and care to the patient's positioning, pressure area care and skin condition.
- Reviewing and maintaining the patient's privacy. Checking comfort and pain control.
- Observation of the patient's condition, appearance, clothing, bed linen and pillows.
- Keeping tidy the patient's immediate bedside environment such as their locker and bedside table.
- Checking that any bedside medical equipment such as oxygen, nebulizers, suction apparatus and intravenous infusions are working efficiently.
- Maintenance and assessment of patients' special daily living aids such as spectacles, hearing aids and walking frames.
- Encouragement of patients to drink fluids and follow their dietary needs.

When carrying out patient comfort rounds, two nurses should work together and cover all the patients on the ward. It is important to use the patient's own toiletries and pay strict attention to infection control guidelines and privacy and dignity. In the past, a trolley was used, laden with laundry and communal equipment such as a bowl, a jug for hot water and various skin lotions and creams. Today, with more individualised patient equipment and toiletries available at the bedside, a clean trolley top with minimal laundry on the bottom shelf and a laundry skip may be all that is needed.

Patients do value regular comfort rounds because it is an opportunity for them to catch up with the nurses, talk through any concerns and freshen themselves up ready for visitors.

All too quickly and frequently the patient's immediate environment becomes messy and littered with bits of equipment. There is a need to check regularly for cleanliness and to remove soiled personal laundry and litter from lockers.

The outcomes of the patient comfort rounds should be discussed and regularly audited with all members of the ward team. Any relevant information should be recorded in the patient's nursing notes or referred to the appropriate support services manager. The areas of nursing care that patient comfort rounds are aimed at improving are:

- general patient hygiene, especially following toileting
- two-hourly changes in the patient position
- mouth care, general skin assessment

- patient observation and charting
- patient comfort
- pain control
- nurse-patient contact
- morale and support.

Like any system of patient nursing care it has to be carefully planned, adopted and reviewed.

Remember what you can do

- Discuss with your colleagues whether you think clinical rounds would be helpful to you and your patients.
- Ask patients and relatives for their views.
- Undertake a pilot of the rounds for a period and audit and evaluate the findings.

References

Castledine G (2002) Patient comfort rounds: a new initiative in nursing. *Br J Nurs* **11**(6): 407

DoH (1989) A Strategy for Nursing: A report from the steering committee. Department of Health Nursing Division, London

DoH (1991) Patient's Charter. Department of Health, London

Chapter 5

Customer care

Ann Close

The old adage 'first impressions are lasting impressions' can never be more true than in the health service. A person's first encounter with a hospital, whether as a patient in the outpatients department, in the emergency department or in a ward or as a visitor, is very likely to colour their perceptions in future. It is therefore extremely important that this first experience is positive. This chapter suggests ways of creating a positive first impression, how to develop effective communication with patients, relatives and others and how to respond to queries and complaints. It also highlights the role of the Patient Advice and Liaison Service (PALS).

People often start to build a picture before they need to use the service. They visit family and friends in hospital, listen to the stories and experiences of others, read about their local hospital in newspapers or have friends and relations who work in the health service. If a patient has had a bad experience they are more likely to tell others about it, and the press are more likely to print the story. The more we can prevent this by improving the service, the better for staff, the hospital and for patients and who will have more confidence in the care they will receive.

Creating a positive first impression

Appointment letters

Most non-emergency patients receive written notification of their hospital appointment or admission. The information they receive should be clear, concise, unambiguous, and courteous and provide all the necessary information about where and when the appointment is, what they should bring with them and who will be seeing them. Most letters will be sent out by health records staff who may not be aware of what patients want to know or if there have been any recent changes. It is therefore important that nursing staff do review these with others from time to time. It can be helpful if you ask patients for their views about the letters.

Telephone contacts

Patients and relatives will often contact the hospital by telephone. It is important that phones are answered quickly. If there are problems because staff are too busy, then alternatives should be considered such as reallocation of duties to ensure someone is available or redirection of calls to someone who can respond. Patients and relatives may be anxious in ringing the hospital for whatever reason and it will be helpful when answering if you:

- are friendly and courteous
- greet the patient with hello or good morning/afternoon
- give your name and department
- ask for the person's name, remember it and use it
- ask how you can help
- deal with the enquiry or, if necessary, give clear instructions on what to do or offer to find out and ring the person back
- make sure no one can over hear your conversation if there is anything of a sensitive or confidential nature
- if you need to leave the caller on hold then you ensure no conversations about other patients can be heard
- make sure patients receive messages from their relatives.

Face-to-face contacts

It is not enough just to turn up to work each day and carry out the various roles and responsibilities. How these are carried out and how you communicate is important.

Meeting and greeting

When a patient, visitor or member of staff arrives in your area the first few seconds are critical to their perception of you and your ward or department.

- Even if you are busy and in the middle of doing something make eye contact, smile, give a greeting and say, 'I'll be with you in a minute'. There is nothing worse than being ignored while the person finishes what they are doing.

- Introduce yourself and ask for their name and how you can help.
- Deal with their enquiry. If they have to wait, make sure they are comfortable and keep them updated about any delays or progress.
- If you have to give instructions, make sure you have communicated them effectively and they are understood.
- If you are asked about a patient you are not looking after that day, provide an initial response to the visitor and then find the nurse who can give a more detailed view. There is nothing more frustrating or upsetting to a relative than being told by the nurse that they don't know because they are 'not one of my patients'.

Similarly if you are in other parts of the hospital and you see people looking lost approach them and ask if you can be of help

Non-verbal cues

Non-verbal communication includes all the ways in which people communicate with each other other than by using words. Facial gestures and body language can demonstrate positive attitudes such as interest, concern and attentiveness or negative attitudes such as boredom, disinterest and impatience. Such non-verbal cues can have a very powerful effect on patients and, no matter what words are used, the message is significantly influenced by these gestures.

Eye contact – you should be looking at the person you are talking to for at least 80% of the conversation. Failure to look at people when you are talking to them and when they are talking to you will stand in the way of successful communication and your developing a positive relationship.

Voice – consider how you sound to others:

- are they able to understand you or do you use technical jargon, a local dialect or speak too softly?
- do you sound interested in them or bored with what you are doing and easily distracted?
- do you sound friendly and caring or are you abrupt or sharp in the way you speak?

Although you may intend to be a sensitive, articulate and effective communicator, an anxious worried patient or relative may not have the same perception. It might be helpful to get some feedback from an honest colleague.

Listening

Effective communication is a two-way process which requires you to actively listen to the patients and not to:

- think of what you want to say in return when the other person is speaking
- finish off sentences for slow speakers
- react to problems before you have all the facts
- let your mind wander to personal problems or other work situations
- assume you know what the person is about to say.

You need to focus on the patient and what they are saying. Check that you have received the correct message by repeating some of the key points or asking questions.

Checking that your message has got through

Many nurses are surprised and upset when patients and relatives complain that they were not given sufficient information or were not told about what was happening to them. This is especially so when they believe that they have provided this information. There have been many studies of communication which show that only about half of all oral instructions are received and retained. Therefore when communicating with patients and relatives you should:

- repeat information as necessary and encourage questions
- remember people tend to filter out unwelcome or bad news and tend to retain positive aspects
- give information in small amounts as people tend to switch off if given too much
- provide the information in writing, where possible, so that patients can read more later.

Addressing others

Make sure that you address people politely. Unless you know them well, you should address them by their title and surname and not with local endearments such as 'love', 'duck' or 'dear' or by their first name. Although these may be intended as friendly, they can actually be offensive to some people.

It is important that staff are easily identified as staff. Uniforms and titles of staff can be very confusing. It is therefore important that you make sure you introduce yourself by name and title and that you wear your name badge or other identification tag. Make sure that you introduce visiting staff such as doctors or therapists if they forget to do this. Having some written information for patients on the staff who are likely to visit them may be helpful too.

Appearance

People do make judgements about each other based on the way they look. Patients and relatives expect certain standards of appearance of all healthcare professionals. If you look untidy, poorly groomed, with an ill fitting or creased uniform, then patients will have the impression that care may also be poor and of a low standard. Although it is fashionable to have 'way out' hairstyles, facial piercing and tattoos, you should remember that these may have a negative impact on some patients and influence their perceptions of you and your care, irrespective of what it is really like. When wearing your uniform remember it should help you display a professional image and it should not put you or the patients' health and safety at risk.

Inappropriate conversations

It is recognised that staff in hospitals are humans with the same sort of worries, concerns and feelings about their personal and work life as any other person. However when they begin to bring these to their working environment and discuss them within the hearing of patients and relatives it is unacceptable as it gives the impression that they are not focused on the work they are doing. It is also inappropriate for staff to complain to patients and relatives about their employer or their dissatisfaction with the health service in general as this undermines the confidence patients have in the service and may be upsetting to them.

Creating lasting impressions

No-one is likely to disagree that first impressions are important but it is essential that positive first impressions are maintained. With the implementation of the Patient Choice initiative (DoH, 2003) it is becoming increasingly important to hospitals that patients see them in a positive light and want to be referred to them for treatment. McIntosh (1997) identified the top ten factors that are likely to lead to patients recommending a hospital to others.

1. Staff sensitivity to the inconvenience that health problems and hospitalisation cause
2. Overall cheerfulness of the hospital
3. Staff concern for patients' privacy
4. Amount of attention paid to patients' special or personal needs
5. Degree to which nurses took patients' health problems seriously
6. Technical skill of nurses
7. Nurses' attitudes to patients calling them
8. Degree to which the nurses kept patients adequately informed about tests, treatment and equipment
9. Friendliness of nurses
10. Promptness in responding to the call button.

Nurse–patient relationships

In addition, an important part of patient care, and therefore customer care, is the relationship between the nurse and the patient. Peplau (1988) suggests that the interpersonal skills of the nurse are the most important part of the nursing role and have more effect on the outcome of a patient's problem that many routine technical procedures. Patients value the opportunity to talk and express their anxieties and have an empathetic nurse who will listen to them. Castledine (2004) recognises that, 'the key to a successful nurse patient relationship is non-judgemental listening and the ability to convey warmth and understanding'. He says the nurse patient relationship is important for ten reasons – to:

- help patients make informal decisions
- avoid isolating and dehumanising patients
- act as an advocate for vulnerable patients and those unable to express their wishes
- nurture co-operation and understanding
- help in patient assessment and problem solving
- help patients cope with their problems
- help patients undertake, or carry out for them, activities of living and human needs
- nurse dying patients and those with terminal illnesses and palliative care needs
- teach and promote health education

- learn about new ways of nursing and caring for people in a changing world.

Responding to queries and complaints

Being in hospital is a stressful time for patients and their relatives. Anxiety about the patient's condition, lack of understanding of what is going on and frustration when information and answers are not readily available may lead to anger, confusion, misunderstandings and confrontations between patients, relatives and nursing staff. When simple concerns are not recognised and dealt with effectively they turn into complaints. Analysis of any hospital's complaints will show that a large proportion of complaints are due to poor communication and that a significant number of other complaints will have poor communication as a component. This is not helpful to anyone but there are ways you can reduce the likelihood of this happening by taking a proactive approach.

Taking a proactive approach may involve:

- Carrying out a round of your patients at the beginning of the shift to:
    - check their condition and make them aware of who is in charge of their care and who they can talk to
    - discuss briefly with each patient their progress and any concerns they may have
    - identify priorities across the group of patients you are responsible for and ensure resources are deployed accordingly
    - monitor care, and ensure documentation and charting is up to date. You can then identify elements of care that have not been completed and that should be passed on to the next shift.
- Having sufficient information about all the patients on your ward so you can respond immediately to enquiries by other members of staff, visiting consultants or to telephone enquiries from the patients' relatives. There is nothing more frustrating than to hear a patient is not your responsibility. If the patient is on your ward they are your responsibility.
- Undertaking rounds at visiting times so that you give the relatives the chance to ask questions without the need to seek you out. You can also ask them if they have any queries or concerns. They may be reluctant to ask or are unsure of whom to approach.
- Making sure that you keep patients up to date with what is happening, for example plans for tests and procedures, transfers and discharges. Remember that patients and their families may need an explanation more than once and that sometimes it will be helpful to give information in writing.

More details on the benefits of these rounds and how to carry them out can be found in *Chapter 4*.

Complaints

It is always disappointing to receive a complaint about the work you do, however, you should try to see it in a positive light in that it has the potential to provide you with an opportunity to improve the services and care you give to patients. If you receive a complaint from a patient or relative you should:

- Try and resolve the complaint as quickly and effectively as possible. It is important that you appear open and not defensive. Discuss your plans and actions with the patient and/or relative and whether they feel this is appropriate and whether any further action needs to take place. You should record the complaint and actions according to your organisation's procedures.
- If the complaint is too complex for you to resolve, or the person complaining wishes to make the complaint formal, then you should contact your complaints manager. You should assist the person concerned by providing telephone numbers and, if necessary, by helping them to write down the substance of their complaint.
- Most organisations have written information about their complaints process and you should ensure that copies are available in your area and that you make them available to patients and their relatives.
- You should make sure that you and your colleagues keep a record of the events relating to the complaint including witness statements.
- You should also make sure that you inform the complaints manager and your line manager of the complaint and that related incidents are recorded if this is the practice in your organisation.
- You should support colleagues who have been complained about and participate in action planning to make changes.
- You should ask for feedback on how the complaint was responded to.

Support from PALS

Patient Advice and Liaison Services were established in 2002 in every NHS organisation. The service are intended to provide on-the-spot help to patients, including:

- advice and support for patients, their families and carers
- information on NHS services

- help to sort out problems quickly
- being there to listen to patients and the public's concerns, suggestions or queries.

PALS acts independently to try and help patients and their families who have concerns and will liaise with staff and managers and others inside and outside the organisation to resolve problems and ultimately to bring about changes in the way services are delivered. PALS will also channel patients to independent advice and advocacy support, including the Independent Complaints Advocacy Service (ICAS) and to other support agencies that may be of help to patients such as the Citizens Advice Bureau and other PALS services, for example in primary care trusts and ambulance services.

PALS also has a role in supporting staff within the organisation and helping them to deal with people more effectively to be more open and to act on feedback received from patients. They are also required to facilitate opportunities for patients, carers and relatives to be involved in decisions about planning and delivering services and about monitoring the quality of services. The philosophy of PALS is that all members of staff have a role to act as a help and support to patients and not to abdicate this role and responsibility to the few individuals in the PALS team. Therefore many PALS teams are involved in training and developing the skills and knowledge of staff and the culture within the organisation.

Remember what you can do

- Consider what first impression you make on others. Ask colleagues for their views.
- Find out what training your organisation has for customer care.
- Discuss with your colleagues their willingness to review and evaluate the customer care in your area.
- Be aware of your organisation's policy and procedures for handling complaints.
- Find out what training there is to help you in handling patients' concerns and complaints and your local PALS.
- Find out what written information on complaints there is available for you to give to patients.
- Keep up to date with national changes to the requirements for complaints' handling.
- Know how to contact your complaints manager.
- Read the Health Service Ombudsman reports on complaints and discuss with your colleagues how you might prevent similar things happening in

your area of work.

■ Contact your PALS team to find out how they work in your organisation and make arrangements to meet with them.

References

Castledine G (2004) The importance of the nurse-patient relationship. *Br J Nurs* **13**(4): 231

Department of Health (2003) Choice of Hospitals, Guidance for PCTs NHS Trusts and SHAs on Offering Patients Choice of Where they are Treated. Department of Health, London

McIntosh T (1997) Empathy: Why patients recommend hospitals. *Healthcare Benchmarks* **4**: 39

Peplau H (1988) Interpersonal Relations in Nursing. MacMillan Education, London

Additional reading

Department of Health (2003) NHS Complaints Reform – Making things Right. DoH, London

Health Service Ombudsman Investigations – produced three times per year

McQueen A (2000) Nurse-patient relationships and partnership in hospital care. *J Clin Nurs* **9**(5): 723–31

Miller L (2002) Effective communication with older people. *Nurs Standard* **17**(19): 45–50, 53, 55

Moore A (2002) Nurse investigator. *Nurs Standard* **17**(9): 12–13

Nursing Standard feature (2002) Facing the Ombudsman. *Nurs Standard* **17**(9) 12–4

Roberts K (2002) Exploring participation: older people on discharge from hospital. *J Adv Nurs* **40**(4): 413–20

Webb B, Brinstead R (2002) Patient panel: an ongoing learning process. *Nurs Standard* **16**(20) 30–42

Useful websites and contacts

www.dh.gov.uk   Department of Health with links to:

■ Commission for Patient and Public Involvement in Health
■ PALS

- Patient and Public Involvement Forum
- ICAS – Independent Complaints Advocacy Service
- NHS direct on-line

www.healthcarecommission.org.uk — Commission for Healthcare Audit and inspection

NHS Direct — Tel: 0845 46 47 operates a 24-hour advice and health information service

Chapter 6

Managing Emergencies

Briony Howells and Amanda Gethin

Emergencies can occur at any time and usually require a rapid response. This chapter highlights the frequently occurring emergencies that happen in hospitals and the general principles that should be followed when they occur. It is essential that you are aware of the policies and procedures in your own organisation so that you can immediately respond if an emergency occurs.

General principles

The following actions are recommended to facilitate the effective management of any situation whether the emergency is of a clinical or non-clinical nature.

- **Don't put yourself at risk**
  Any potential harm or risk to yourself may result in your not being able to help others. It is important to think and make an initial plan rapidly before you act.
- **Keep calm**
  Adrenaline levels may be raised but you should maintain a calm and professional manner. This in turn will instil confidence in those around you: patients, relatives and staff members. Staying calm will help you to adopt a rational and logical approach to the emergency.
- **Acknowledge your own limitations**
  If you are lacking in the skills, knowledge or expertise to deal with a situation, do not be afraid to seek help, guidance and support from other sources, such as your line manager, colleagues, senior nurse, manager on call, specialist nurses or medical staff.
- **Reassurance and explanation**
  It is important to remember that patients will be frightened and anxious, therefore offering them reassurance and an explanation of what is happening is a vital part of the care and relevant in the management of conscious and unconscious patients alike.

- **Attendance at mandatory lectures**
  It is every individual's responsibility to ensure they attend a fire, manual handling and cardio-pulmonary resuscitation update, annually. The knowledge and skills you gain will help you in the appropriate management of the emergency.
- **Knowledge of trust/hospital policies**
  Use policies as a reference to guide you in dealing with a situation. No one is expected to know the policies word for word, but you should have a good overall understanding of the key points. It is important you know where to access the policy relevant to the emergency/situation.
- **Maintenance of equipment**
  Equipment should be checked and serviced regularly, eg daily checks of oxygen and suction equipment. Any equipment not working should be taken out of service and reported immediately according to your trust/ hospital policy. Using vital equipment may be essential to the effective management of an emergency situation.
- **Completion of adverse incident forms**
  The reporting of an adverse incident either clinical or non-clinical highlights both effective actions and problems experienced during the emergency and therefore the need to reassess and, at times, change practice and procedures. It may also highlight the need for training. Appropriate action will in turn assist in the prevention and reduction of incidents of a similar nature .

Clinical emergencies

Harrison and Daly (2001) believe that the basis for effective care during a medical emergency must be a clear understanding by the nurse of the underlying medical condition. Everything else they state, 'follows on from this: a logical approach to initial assessment; appropriate monitoring, timely and effective emergency care and the anticipation of potential complications'.

Patient assessment

The systematic approach adopted when undertaking the immediate assessment of any clinical emergency follows the mnemonic ABCDE, as follows:

Table 6.1		
A	Airway	• speak to the patient; ask them if they are all right. If the patient responds appropriately there is unlikely to be an airway problem • look, listen and feel for expired air • maintain airway with a jaw thrust or chin lift • place the patient in the recovery position providing there is no evidence of an injury to the spine • if tolerated use a guedel oral airway • administer high-flow oxygen
B	Breathing	• count the respiratory rate • listen for noise • assess the effort • perform oximetry • administer high-flow oxygen • monitor oxygen saturation
C	Circulation	• assess pulse rate and strength and volume • assess capillary refill • measure the blood pressure
D	Disability	• check conscious level • assess Glasgow Coma Scale • assess pupil size, equality and reaction
E	Exposure	• perform full body check of the patient • look for any abnormalities, eg deformity or rashes

Many different clinical emergencies can present in any system of the body. It is important, therefore, to remember that while the management may differ, the immediate assessment follows the same logical approach as identified above.

The following are examples of the immediate nursing management, observations and care administered to the more frequently encountered clinical emergencies within a medical setting.

Cardio-respiratory arrest

On finding an unresponsive patient, you should rapidly assess the situation, (using ABC) and, if required, commence basic life support:

Immediate management/observations

■ Ensure that the area surrounding the patient is safe and there are no stray wires or water on the floor. This prevents you and others causing harm to yourselves, or further harm to the patient.

■ Assess whether the patient is responsive: call their name.

■ Check the patient's airway for any obvious obstruction.

- Call for assistance.
- Watch the patient's chest for movement. Listen and feel at the patient's mouth for breath sounds (10 seconds).
- Administer two breaths.
- Feel for the carotid pulse (10 seconds) - if the pulse is absent alert the cardiac arrest team.
- Continue the resuscitation procedure according to your organisation's resuscitation policy.

Subsequent management/observations

- Secure venous access.
- Delegate staff not involved in CPR to screen the emergency from other patients.
- Ensure the patient's record is available for medical and other staff.
- Infection control and health and safety principles should be maintained.
- Contact the patient's relatives.
- Ensure the patient's condition is closely monitored (this is obviously dependent on the success of the resuscitation attempt).
- Do not leave the patient unattended.
- Keep accurate records of the event in the nursing record with details of timing.

Chest pain and angina

Any patient who complains of chest pain must be investigated immediately.

The patient may present with breathlessness, pallor, sweating, hypotension, nausea or vomiting and appear distressed.

Immediate management/observations

- ABC assessment.
- Monitor oxygen saturation – they may require oxygen therapy.
- Record blood pressure and pulse.
- Record or request an urgent ECG – to rule out a myocardial infarction or angina.
- Reassure the patient.
- Summon medical assistance.

The nurse should also ask the patient the following:

- describe the pain

- where is the pain?
- does it radiate anywhere?
- how long have they had the pain?
- what, if anything, makes it worse?

Subsequent management/observations

- Secure venous access.
- Administer prescribed pain relief.
- Assess effectiveness of the pain relief.
- Monitor blood pressure and pulse regularly.
- Care for intravenous infusions.
- Make accurate and timely records.
- Give explanations to the patient and family as appropriate.

Acute asthmatic attack

Immediate management/observations

- ABC assessment.
- Monitor and record the following:
  - respiratory rate (abnormal respiratory rate >25 breaths per minute)
  - pulse rate (abnormal > 110 beats per minute)
  - peak expiratory flow (PEF) (abnormal < 50%)
  - oxygen saturation (abnormal< 92%)
  - the inability to complete a sentence in one breath
  - summon medical attention immediately.

NB It is important to be aware that patients with severe or life-threatening attacks may not be distressed or experience all, or even any, of the above abnormal observations. In fact they may have normal oxygen saturation, may be calmer and co-operative before suffering a respiratory arrest.

Subsequent management/observation

- Give reassurance and support.
- Secure venous access.

- Explain to the patient the management of their condition.
- Sit patient upright. The patient will find the most comfortable position for themselves eg leaning over a bed table, sitting on the edge of the bed.
- Administer prescribed oxygen. In the event that none is prescribed, then check if there is a local policy which will allow administration of oxygen in such circumstances. Administer prescribed nebuliser therapy.
- Monitor oxygen saturation via pulse oximetry.
- Assist medical staff with the administration of intravenous medications.
- Monitor the patient's response to treatment.
- Record peak expiratory flow if the patient is able.
- Record the pulse rate every fifteen minutes for the first hour.
- Complete documentation.

Upper gastro-intestinal haemorrhage

Patients with major gastro-intestinal bleeding need instant assessment and urgent resuscitation (Harrison and Daly, 2001).

Immediate management/observations

- ABC assessment.
- Summon immediate medical attention.
- Ensure the safety of the patient.
- Administer oxygen therapy.
- Secure venous access (restore circulation volume).
- Observe for signs of shock.
- Monitor blood pressure, pulse and respirations (quarter to half-hourly), record all observations (tachycardia, hypotension, clammy skin, pallor, confusion and restlessness).

Subsequent management/observations

- Reassure the patient.
- Explain procedures.
- Chart all blood loss.
- Keep an accurate fluid balance chart (catheterise patient).
- Monitor and record blood pressure and pulse regularly.
- Care of intravenous infusions.
- Complete documentation.

Fits and seizures

Immediate management/observations

- ABCDE assessment.
- Of prime importance is the safety of the patient. Protect them from harm but don't try to hold on to the patient when they are thrashing about.
- Do not place anything in the patient's mouth during a seizure.
- Administer high flow of oxygen.
- Secure venous access.
- Summon medical assistance.

Subsequent management/observations

- Protect the airway (when more relaxed, attempt to insert a guedel airway).
- Only when the seizure has ceased place the patient in the recovery position (it may cause injury if they are moved during the seizure).
- Check for any injuries which may have been sustained during the time of the seizure.
- Reassure and explain to the patient what happened.
- Administer intravenous medication prescribed by the medical staff.
- Observe for respiratory depression.
- Do not leave the patient unattended until they are fully recovered.
- Complete documentation.

Diabetic ketoacidosis

When caring for a patient who has been diagnosed with diabetic ketoacidosis (DKA), the nurse should recognise that the first few hours of treatment and care are critical.

The patient may appear confused, dehydrated, and distressed.

Immediate management/observations

- ABC assessment.
- Monitor oxygen saturation.

- Record blood pressure and pulse rate.
- Venous access.
- Record blood sugar.

Subsequent management/observations

- Record or request ECG.
- Monitor blood sugar–BM recordings hourly.
- Test urine for ketones.
- Catheterise if necessary.
- Obtain MSU (midstream specimen of urine).
- Record accurate fluid balance.
- Record temperature and observe for signs of infection.
- Monitor respiratory rate.
- Record Glasgow coma score (see table 6.2 below).
- Provide reassurance for the patient and family.
- Accurately record observations.
- Care for the intravenous infusion.
- Complete documentation.
- Continue to monitor patient closely.

Table 6.2: Glasgow coma score

The Glasgow coma score is the universal measurement of the depth of coma. The scores reflect the severity of the neurological status:
Mild: 13 to 15
Moderate: 9 to 12
Severe: 3 to 8

Response	Score
Eye opening	
spontaneously	4
to verbal command	3
to pain	2
no response	1
Best motor response	
obeys commands	6
localises to pain	5
withdraws to pain	4
abnormal flexion to pain	3
extension to pain	2
no response	1
Best verbal response	
orientated and converses	5
disorientated and converses	4
inappropriate words	3
incomprehensible	2
no response	
Total score (3 to 15)	

Hypoglycaemia

On finding a patient who has impaired consciousness, neurological or behavioural disturbances consider the possibility of hypoglycaemia.

The patient may present with sweating, changes in their behaviour, tremor and complain of palpitations.

Immediate management/observations

- ABC assessment.
- Record blood sugar–BM reading.
- Record blood pressure and pulse.
- If conscious and able to swallow, give 25 grams of glucose in 150 mls of water to drink.
- If patient is unconscious:
  - Secure airway
  - Secure venous access
- Seek immediate medical assistance.

Subsequent management/observations

- Monitor blood sugar–BM recordings hourly.
- Nurse in recovery position.
- Closely monitor the patient during unconsciousness.
- Provide reassurance for the patient and family.
- Explain the event to the patient.
- Complete documentation.

Non-clinical situations

The following are examples of non-clinical emergencies or situations that may be encountered and require action to be taken.

Patient absconded from the ward or unit

- Search the ward/unit area thoroughly.
- Inform security staff and work with them to search the hospital. Provide a description of the patient.
- Inform medical staff.
- Inform duty manager, senior nurse or equivalent.
- Contact the patient's relatives.

- Consider the need to ask police for their assistance. You will need to provide them with a description of the patient and details of their home.
- Discuss with the medical staff whether the patient needs to return to hospital to continue treatment.
- Complete an adverse incident form.
- Document the event in the patients nursing process.

Fire

Hospitals are particularly vulnerable to fire because of the risks associated with special processes, electrical equipment and medical gas supplies. Because of the danger it is essential that all staff understand what is required of them, and to co-operate effectively to ensure patient, visitor and staff safety in the event of fire. You must therefore regard fire precaution as a basic duty. You should:

- Ensure you are aware of the details of your fire policy.
- Check whom you inform in the case of, or suspicion of, a fire and how you do this. Usually it includes
  - sounding the alarm
  - dialling 2222 to inform switchboard the fire is in your area
  - or contacting the emergency fire services directly.
- Ensure you are aware of the fire alarm and exit points in your area of work.
- Ensure you are aware of the different patterns of alarm and what they mean, eg continuous alarm and intermittent alarm.
- Ensure you know what fire fighting equipment is available in your area, what it is used for and how to use it.
- Ensure you know your role in the procedure for evacuation, what you should instruct others to do and where the evacuation point is for your ward or department.
- You should also make sure that new staff working in the area are made aware of these procedures.
- Make sure you attend a fire lecture at least every year to remind yourself of the principles and to learn any new procedures.
- If the fire is in your area, you have alerted the fire services and summoned help from within the hospital you should:
  - remove any patient who is in immediate danger to a safer place, eg behind fire doors
  - assess its severity and tackle only if safe to do so
  - ensure fire doors and windows are closed
  - switch off all equipment unless it would put the patient in danger to do so
  - be aware of all staff, patients and others on your area at the time

- instruct staff to evacuate patients if appropriate. Usually ambulant patients should be moved first
- reassure the patients and keep them fully aware of the situation
- report to the Fire Service Officer any patient, visitor or staff member who you cannot account for
- under no circumstances should any patient, visitor or member of staff return to the area until told it is safe to do so by the Fire Service Officer.

- If the fire is not in your area you should:
  - be able to send help to other areas according to your policy.
  - restrict the movement of patients, visitors and staff to your ward or department until the all clear is given.

Utility failure

An emergency situation will occur if there is:

- mains power failure – equipment, lighting and telecommunications
- water failure
- medical gases failure including suction
- equipment Group failure eg all drug fridges, or individual items that are unique to an area.

Fortunately, failure of water and medical gases is relatively rare. Electricity failure is not unknown but the majority of hospitals have a generator back-up system that starts within seconds of the failure of the mains supply. In your ward and department you should be aware of the contingency plans in place to cope with such a utility failure and what action you need to take to prevent injury and harm to patients, staff and visitors. This may include:

- obtaining emergency supplies such as head torches and batteries in the event of lighting failure
- using electrically operated beds if power fails
- acting to conserve energy in partial power failure
- using manual alternatives to electrically operated equipment, eg portable or battery suction units, manual sphygmomanometers.
- using arrangements for communication, with doctors, managers and others, are there special 'fall back phones', mobile phones, will battery-operated bleeps continue to work for short periods?
- making arrangements to be taken for toilet provision, personal hygiene and drinking water in the case of water failure.

Remember what you can do

As a trained nurse you may be the person in charge of a team of nurses and responsible for a ward of patients and even their visitors. Remembering the following will help you

Try to keep calm. This will help others and help you think.
Keep up to date with training on all emergency procedures: you never know when you will have to use them.
Keep up to date with all policies relating to emergency situations.
Remember the mnemonic ABCDE and the actions you need to take.

References

Carrison R, Daly L (2001) Acute Medical Emergencies: A Nursing Guide. Churchill Livingstone, London

Additional reading

Black S (1999) A race against time. Nurs Standard **13**(21): 10–6 February: 24–5
Tioffi J (2000) Recognition of patients who require emergency assistance: a descriptive study. *Heart and Lung. J Acute Crit Care* **29**(4): 262–8
Harrison S (2002) Less than ready. *Nurs Standard* **17**(11): 12–3
evon P (2002) Resuscitation in hospital: Resus Council UK recommendations *Nurs Standard* **16**(33): 41–4
McMahon B, Buswell K, Mellors D, Hehir B (2002) An emergency call. *Nurs Standard* **16**(48): 20–1
earce L (2002) Always on the case. *Nurs Standard* **16**(42): 16–7

Helpful websites

www.dh.gov.uk	Department of Health – Emergency Planning
www.emergency-nurse.com	Emergency nursing resource

Chapter 7

Wound management

Gill Hiskett

There have been dramatic changes in wound management over the past ten years with an increase in the scientific approach to wound healing. The development of 'intelligent dressings' and a variety of innovative wound management therapies leaves today's nurse with a bewildering choice of treatment options. This chapter defines the different types of wound and describes the stages of wound healing, wound assessment and the importance of assessment in prevention.

Background

Wound assessment has traditionally been the responsibility of the nurse and often said to be subjective rather than based on best-published evidence to support such practice.

Effective wound management depends on accurate wound assessment, and includes identifying problems and using objective methods of measurement before application of dressing treatments. (Williams, 2000).

In today's society we see an increase in the number of complaints and amount of litigation particularly in respect of chronic wounds such as pressure ulcers and must therefore ensure that wound management incorporates accurate wound assessment and documentation of the findings of that assessment.

What is a wound ?

A wound may be defined as a 'break in the continuity of the skin' and is categorised as either acute or chronic depending upon the cause.

Acute wounds

Acute wounds are usually due to surgical incision or trauma. The aim of treatment is to align the wound edges and to promote complete healing without any secondary problems such as infection.

Acute wounds heal by primary intention.

Chronic wounds

Chronic wounds are said to be wounds that fail to progress past the inflammatory phase of the healing process (University of Dundee, 1993). Chronic wounds, eg pressure ulcers, leg ulcers, are complex wounds and are affected by a range of intrinsic (eg diabetes, rheumatoid arthritis) and extrinsic (eg pressure, friction, shear) factors.

These wounds are seen as open wounds, which aim to heal by secondary intention.

The aim of treatment is to reduce the size of the wound or complete healing.

Clinicians who are involved in wound care should have an understanding of the processes involved in wound healing and the factors that may delay that process. This will allow them to identify what stage of the healing process the wound is at and to make appropriate decisions on the management of that wound.

Stages of wound healing

From the moment a wound is created, the healing process commences. There is much cellular activity involved and, although different phases of the healing process are identified, the activity involved in each phase overlaps.

- inflammatory phase
- destructive phase
- proliferative phase
- maturation/re-modelling phase.

Wound assessment

The aim of wound assessment is to provide the practitioner with baseline information so that an informed decision can be made on the management of that wound including dressing selection and /or equipment selection. Initial assessment should be made at the time of the admission. Further assessment is necessary during the patient's stay, dictated by the needs of the wound, to allow the clinician to monitor the progress of the wound and make changes to the programme of care as necessary. Wound assessment should include the following although the list is not exhaustive:

Patient holistic assessment

- age
- height/weight
- disease
- medication
- psychological state
- social needs
- nutrition
- continence
- mobility
- smoker/non-smoker
- past medical history
- previous surgery
- family history of disease
- allergies.

Wound assessment

- type of wound
- position on the body
- is there undermining?
- structures involved eg tendon, bone.

Size

- maximum length

- maximum width
- maximum depth.

Tissue type

- % necrotic tissue (black)
- % sloughy tissue (yellow)
- % granulation tissue (red)
- % epithelialising tissue (pink).

Exudate

- amount (high, medium, low)
- consistency
- colour
- odour.

Surrounding skin

- healthy
- macerated
- oedema
- erythema (redness)
- eczema
- dry/scaling.

Pain

- type
- duration
- when eg. at dressing changes.

Malodour

- is it present?

Signs of infection

- pus
- increase in pain
- friable tissue
- bridging
- abnormal smell
- cellulitis
- increase in exudate
- delayed healing
- increase in malodour
- wound breakdown.

(Cutting and Harding, 1994)

Chronic wounds (leg ulcers, pressure ulcers) require more in-depth assessment due to their complexity, to ensure that the management is appropriate.

Specific wound assessment – leg ulceration

A leg ulcer has been defined as, 'a loss of skin below the knee on the leg or foot which takes more than six weeks to heal.' (Dale et al, 1983).

Leg ulceration affects around 580,000 people in the UK with 1–2 % of the population affected at any one time (DoH, 1989), with the cost to the NHS estimated at being about £300–£600 million per annum.

The most common cause of leg ulceration is venous disease accounting for 70% of all leg ulcers (Cornwall et al, 1986, Callum et al, 1987). Other aetiologies include arterial disease, diabetes and vasculitis.

In order to provide the appropriate management of the leg ulcer, it is essential that a comprehensive accurate assessment is carried out so that accurate diagnosis can be achieved.

Previously, clinicians have been criticised for their assessment techniques. Poor assessment can lead to inaccurate diagnosis, inappropriate treatments, wasted nursing effort and NHS funds. Ultimately, the patient's wound healing journey will be ongoing.

If an assessment follows a pre-planned structure, it is more likely that the patient will receive appropriate treatment. Comprehensive leg ulcer assessment documentation should be completed for each presenting leg ulcer patient.

Assessment of the leg ulcer patient will include:

- holistic assessment
- limb assessment
- wound assessment.

Holistic assessment

It is important to identify any intrinsic or extrinsic factors that may have an influence on the healing process and that may assist the clinician in accurate diagnosis.

- social history
- age, sex
- mobility
- nutritional status
- disease (eg diabetes, circulatory disorder, rheumatoid arthritis)
- medication
- family history of ulcers
- history of smoking
- vascular history
- pregnancy
- previous history of ulceration.

Limb assessment

- visible varicosities
- size
- shape
- evidence of previous ulceration, trauma, surgery
- brown discoloration (veinous staining)
- dependency colour changes(palor on elevation)
- oedema, cellulites
- phlebitis
- skin type (fragile, scaly)
- atrophy blanche (white stippled with red)
- lipodermatosclerosis (hard, woody)
- shiny tight skin
- trophic changes in the nails
- ankle mobility.

Ulcer assessment

- site
- size
- ulcer history (trauma?)
- duration of ulcer
- clinical signs of infection
- exudate (odour, consistency, colour, amount)
- pain (severity, when, type)
- surrounding skin (inflammation, maceration, discolouration)
- stage of wound healing (% of necrotic tissue, slough, granulation).

Doppler

Historically, the presence of pedal pulses identified by palpitation has been used in the diagnosis and aetiology of the ulcer. However this has proven to be unreliable (Moffatt and O'Hare, 1995). Barnhorst and Barner (1968) noted that up to 12% of the population had absent dorsalis pedis pulses and stated that oedema of the limb can make palpitation of the pulses difficult.

Clinical assessment has proved to be inaccurate in about one third of cases and therefore the use of a hand-held, mini Doppler ultrasound to assist with diagnosis is an important part of the assessment process. The aim is to measure the arterial flow to the limb by calculating the ankle brachial pressure index (ABPI). This procedure should only be carried out by first level nurses who are trained and competent in carrying it out.

The assessment of leg ulceration is complex and time consuming. With accurate assessment and an appropriate treatment regime, the ulceration may heal without complication or delay.

Pressure ulcers

Defined as:

> *A new or established area of skin and or tissue discolouration or damage which persists after the removal of pressure and which is likely to be due to the effects of pressure on the tissue*

(DoH, 1993).

Pressure ulcers (pressure sores, bed sores) are not a new problem as they have been in existence for decades. Florence Nightingale (1861) proposed that good nursing care could prevent pressure ulcers. But does this mean that they are due to poor nursing care?

Today, through scientific research we understand that pressure ulcers develop due to a combination of factors: pressure shear, friction (extrinsic factors) and a variety of pathophysiological conditions (intrinsic factors) such as disease, age, reduced mobility, incontinence, poor nutrition and mental alertness.

Pressure ulcers undoubtedly cause considerable pain and suffering and often increase patients' hospital stay. In some instances they are stated as the causative factor of death.

The true financial cost to the NHS is unknown but it is estimated to be in excess of £60 million per annum (DoH, 1991).

It is commonly thought that most pressure ulcers are preventable. Waterlow (1988) suggested that 95% were preventable, however intervention for prevention can be expensive. It is important, therefore, to ensure that the limited resources available are used appropriately by carrying out an accurate assessment of need. To identify patients at risk of developing pressure damage, it is necessary to undertake an assessment of that risk level by using a formal structured assessment process.

In the prevention and management of pressure ulcers, the importance of assessment tools is growing, particularly in today's climate of financial constraint, limited resources and the fear of litigation.

There are a variety of 'risk' assessment tools that have been developed since the 1950s. All have been found to have limitations in their predictive value and yet are widely used. The 'Waterlow Risk Assessment' tool is the most commonly used of the tools.

Pressure ulcer risk assessment should be carried out according to your organisation's policy. Commonly this recommend initial assessment within two hours of admission and reassessment according to the patient's dependency rating.

Waterlow Risk Assessment tool considers the intrinsic and extrinsic factors associated with the aetiology and pathogenesis of pressure ulcers.

Table 7.1: Waterlow risk assessment	Initials														
	Date														
Response	**No.**	1	2	3	4	5	6	7	8	9	10	11	12	13	14
Body weight for height															
average	0														
above average	1														
obese	2														
below average	3														
Continence															
completely	0														
occasionally	1														
cath, incontinence or faeces	2														
doubly incontinent	3														
Skin type – visual risk areas															
healthy	0														
tissue paper dry	1														
oedematous clammy (temp T)	1														
discoloured	2														
broken spot	3														
Mobility															
fully	0														
restless/fidgety	1														
apethetic	2														
restricted	3														
inert/traction	4														
chairbound	5														
Age/sex															
Male/female	½														
14–49	1														
50–64	2														
65–74	3														
75–80	4														
80+	5														

Table 7.1: Waterlow risk assessment	Initials														
	Date														
Response	**No.**	1	2	3	4	5	6	7	8	9	10	11	12	13	14
Appetite															
average	0														
poor	1														
NG tubes/fluids only	2														
NBM/anorexic	3														
Special risks – tissue mal.															
terminal/cachexia	3														
cardiac failure	5														
peripheral vascular disease	5														
anaemia	2														
smoking	1														
Neurological defects															
diabetes, MS, CVA	4–6														
motor sensory paraplegia															
Major surgery/trauma															
orthopaedic	5														
below waist/spinal	5														
on table over 2 hours	5														
Medications															
cytoxics, highdose steroids	4														
anti-inflammatory															
Total score															

7.1 Waterlow Risk Assessment (1988),
first published in *Care – Science and Practice*, reproduced by permission.

It is essential to consider the patient's skin condition and, in conjunction with the Waterlow risk assessment, identify any existing tissue damage. Particular attention should be paid to the known susceptible areas of the body.

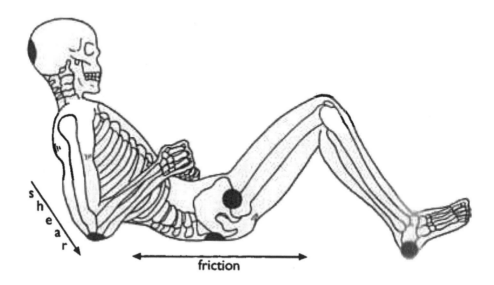

● major points of pressure over bony prominences

⟶ 'forces' acting on skin

friction

Figure 7.1 Shear and friction can also cause damage

Existing tissue damage should be assessed in accordance with the organisation's policy. A recommended assessment grading tool is from the Agency for Health Care Policy and Research (1994)

Table 7.2: Pressure sore grading tool (AHCPR, 1994)	
Grade 1	Descolouration of intact skin, including non blanchable erythema. Non blancable erythema – erythema remains under light finger pressue indicating damage to micro circulation.
Grade 2	Partial thickness skin loss or damage involving the epidermis and/or dermis.
Grade 3	Full thickness skin loss involving damage or necrosis of subcutaneous tissue, but not through the underlaying fascia and not extending to the underlying bone, tendon or joint capsule.
Grade 4	Full thickness skin loss with extensive destruction and tissue necrosis extending to the underlying bone, tendon or joint capsule.

The information obtained in the assessment process will assist the clinician to develop an appropriate management strategy for the patient including appropriate selection of pressure reducing/relieving equipment.

Table 7.3: Pressure damage				
Waterlow score/equipment	Gr 1	Gr 2	Gr 3	Gr 4
High/very high 20+ 　eg Nimbusil + seating				
Medium 15–19 + seating 　eg Autoexcell				
Low 10–14 + seating 　eg Alphaexcell				
At risk > 10 　eg Softfoam/Transform Propad + seating				
Comfort 　Fibre-filled mattress overlay eg Spenco Super down				

Conclusion

Accurate wound assessment is an important factor in the management of wounds. The assessment process should be undertaken by a first level nurse, who has the relevant knowledge and skills and who is competent in carrying out this procedure. Accurate assessment of a wound will enable the practitioner to identify any factors that may contribute to a delay in the wound healing process and to make an informed decision on the most appropriate wound products/ therapies to be used.

Remember what you can do

- Ensure you are up to date in how to assess wounds.
- Ensure you are up to date with policies and standards in your organisation for assessing wounds.
- Ensure you know which pressure sore risk assessment tool is used and that you are able to use it in practice to identify the type of equipment you should be using for each patient.
- Ensure you can grade pressure sores.
- Seek help and advice from your tissue viability nurse specialist.

References

Agency for Health Care Policy and Research (1994) Treatment of Pressure Ulcers: Clinical Practice Guideline No. 15. AHCPR, USA

Barnhorst DA, Barner HB (1968) Prevalence of Congenitally absent Pedal Pulses. N Engl J Med 278: 264–5

Callam MJ, Harper DR, Dale JJ, Ruckley CV (1987) Chronic ulcer of the leg: clinical history. *Br Med J* **294**(6584): 1389–91

Cornwall JV, Dore CJ, Lewis JD (1986) Leg ulcers; epidemiology and aetiology. *Br J Surg* **73**: 693–6

Cutting K, Harding K (1994) Criteria for identifying wound infection. *J Wound Care* **3**(4): 198–201

Dale J, Callam M, Ruckley C, Harper D, Berrey P (1983) Chronic ulcers of the leg: a study of prevalence in a Scottish community. *Health Bulletin* **41**: 310–4

DoH (1989) Gravitational (Varicose) Ulcers: The Problem, What we Know and What we Need to Know and Do. Seminar, 30 November, DoH. HMSO, London

DoH (1991)The Health of the Nation. HMSO, London

DoH (1993) Pressure Sores: a Key Quality Indicator. HMSO, London

Moffatt C, O'Hare L (1995) Ankle pulses are not sufficient to detect impaired arterial circulation in patients with leg ulcers. *J Wound Care* **4**(3): 14–8

Nightingale F, (1861) Notes on Nursing. Appleton Century, New York

Torrance (1990) Sleep and wound healing. *Surg Nurs* **3**(3): 16–20

University of Dundee (1993) The Wound Programme (1993) Centre for Medical Education, University of Dundee.

Waterlow J (1988) The Waterlow card for the prevention and management of pressure sores –towards a pocket policy. *Care Sci Pract* **6**(1): 8–12

Williams C (2000) The verge videometer wound management package. *Br J Nurs* **9**(4): 237–9

Additional reading

Tissue Viability Supplements. *Br J Nursing* **11**(20), **12**(11), **12**(15), **12**(19), **13**(15)

Useful websites

www.ewma.org — European Wound Management Association

www.internurse.com — On-line archive peer reviewed articles

www.diabeticfootjournal.com	Diabetic Foot Journal, Journal of Diabetes Nursing, Diabetes Digest, Diabetes and Primary Care
www.tvs.org.uk	Tissues Viability Society
www.tvna.org.uk	Tissue Viability Nurse Association
www.smtl.co.uk/world-wide-wounds	World Wide Wounds
www.etrs.org	European Tissue Repair Society
www.journalofwoundcare.com	Journal of Wound Care
www.epuap.org	European Pressure Ulcer Advisory Panel

Chapter 8

The interpretation of laboratory data

Mourad Labib and Sally Labib

Laboratories offer an extensive and ever-growing repertoire of tests. You should become familiar with tests that are frequently requested in your area. It is always prudent to seek the advice of the laboratory when results do not seem appropriate in the clinical context. This chapter describes the commonest laboratory tests used and the causes of abnormal results. Reference ranges can vary between laboratories and it is important to always check reference ranges with your local laboratory.

The chapter is divided into three sections

- Clinical biochemistry
- Haematology
- Microbiology.

and the tests are in alphabetical order.

Clinical biochemistry

Biochemical tests, either singly or collectively (eg. renal profile), are useful in monitoring disease processes. Although the majority of tests are not specific for any particular condition, they provide sufficient information to indicate the nature of a patient's illness and the direction for further investigations.

Albumin (plasma)

Albumin is synthesised solely in the liver and is the major plasma protein. It is the most important determinant of plasma oncotic pressure (osmotic pressure due to protein) and therefore the distribution of fluid between the vascular and interstitial spaces. It is also involved in the transport of numerous substances including unconjugated bilirubin, calcium, hormones, metals and drugs.

Reference range:	35–50 g/L
Specimen:	whole blood

Causes of low albumin	Causes of high albumin
Poor nutrition Chronic liver disease Hypercatabolic states (sepsis, malignancy) Loss from gut (Crohn's, ulcerative colitis) Loss from kidneys (nephritic syndrome) Overhydration (iatrogenic: inappropriate IV fluids)	Dehydration

Useful tips

- The plasma half-life of albumin is 15–21 days. This may explain why, in fulminant liver failure or acute hepatitis, albumin may initially be normal.
- About 50% of calcium is bound to albumin and therefore a low albumin will result in low serum calcium. However, in this situation, the free ionised (active) calcium is normal.
- About 25% of magnesium is bound to albumin and a very low albumin (<25 g/L) will give a falsely low serum magnesium.

Alkaline phosphatase (ALP)

ALP is mainly present in the liver and bone. Therefore, increased plasma activity occurs in liver and bone diseases.

Reference range (adults):	25–120 IU/L
(children):	up to three times the adult range
Specimen:	whole blood

Causes of high ALP	Causes of low ALP

Bone disease:
  Bone tumours (secondary or primary)
  Fractures (healing)
  Osteomalacia and rickets
  Osteomyelitis
  Paget's disease of bone
  Primary hyperparathyroidism
  Renal osteodystrophy
Liver disease:
  Biliary obstruction
  Cholangitis
  Cirrhosis
  Hepatic tumours (secondary or primary)
	Congenital hypophosphatasia.

Useful tips

- When the origin of high ALP is in doubt, a high GGT (see later) may suggest a liver origin, whereas an abnormal serum calcium may indicate a bony origin. Also, the laboratory should be able to measure bone ALP isoenzyme separately.
- Up to a three-fold increase may be seen in adolescence (bone origin) and pregnancy (placental type).
- An isolated increase in ALP of liver origin may indicate the presence of a 'space-occupying lesion'.

Alanine transaminase (ALT)

ALT is widely distributed in body tissues but is present in high amounts in the liver. It is released into the circulation when there is cell damage as in hepatitis.

Reference range:	0–45 IU/L
Specimen:	whole blood

Causes of high ALT	Causes of low ALT
Cirrhosis Cholestasis Hepatic congestion (congestive cardiac failure) Hepatocellular damage (e.g. viral hepatitis, paracetamol overdose)	Low levels are uncommon and are rarely of any consequence.

Amylase

Amylase is primarily produced by the pancreas and salivary glands. Its measurement is indicated in patients presenting with acute abdominal pain.

Reference range:	0–120 IU/L
Specimen:	whole blood

Causes of high amylase	Causes of low amylase
Acute pancreatitis (usually 3 times the upper limit of reference range) Intestinal obstruction Intestinal infarction Ectopic pregnancy Pelvic inflammatory disease Pancreatic carcinoma Renal insufficiency Diabetic ketoacidosis Opiate use Parotitis Macroamylasaemia	Low levels are of no significance

Useful tips

- Macroamylasaemia is a benign condition in which amylase is complexed with an immunoglobulin giving a high serum level. Because of the low renal clearance of the complex, urine amylase is normal.
- Severe hypertriglyceridaemia interferes with serum amylase measurement and may give false low values in acute pancreatitis. The measurement of urine amylase (amylase/creatinine clearance ratio) is important to make the diagnosis in these cases.
- Measurement of amylase is of no value in the diagnosis of either chronic pancreatic insufficiency or pancreatic cancer.

Aspartate transaminase (AST)

AST is widely distributed in body tissues, particularly in the liver, striated muscle (skeletal and cardiac), red cells, brain, kidneys and lungs.

Reference range:	0–55 IU/L
Specimen:	whole blood

Causes of high AST	Causes of low AST
Liver disease: hepatocellular damage (eg viral hepatitis, paracetamol overdose), cirrhosis, cholestasis and hepatic congestion (congestive cardiac failure). Elevations up to 1-2 times the upper limit of reference range can occur with excessive alcohol intake, obesity, diabetes mellitus and as side effects of many common drugs. Myocardial infarction: Levels rise 12-18 hours after the onset of chest pain and may remain elevated for 3 days. Skeletal muscle: myositis, rhabdomyolysis and myopathy.	Low levels are uncommon and are rarely of any consequence

Useful tips:

- Haemolysed samples can give erroneous results.
- If AST is elevated but other liver tests are normal and there are no clinical features of liver disease, creatine kinase (CK) should be measured to exclude a muscle source.

Bilirubin

Bilirubin is the end product of haem degradation. It is a yellow-orange pigment, which is normally metabolised in the liver and then excreted into the bile. Jaundice usually only becomes apparent when serum bilirubin is at least two to three times the upper normal.

Reference range:	0–17 μmol/L
Specimen:	whole blood

Causes of high biliruin	Causes of low bilirubin
Biliary obstruction Cirrhosis (advanced) Hepatitis (not initially) Hepatic metastases Pancreatic carcinoma Congestive cardiac failure (hepatic congestion) Drug reactions Gilbert's disease Haemolytic conditions	None

Useful tips

■ The urine does not normally contain bilirubin. Bilirubinuria is always pathological.
■ In a jaundiced patient, the presence of bilirubin in urine indicates hepatobiliary disease.
■ In haemolytic conditions, there is no bilirubin in urine and the serum bilirubin rarely exceeds 100 µmol/L.

Blood Gases

Arterial blood gas analysis typically measures:

• pH (a measure of acidity or alkalinity of the blood)
• pCO_2 (partial pressure of carbon dioxide)
• pO_2 (partial pressure of oxygen).
• base excess (the loss of buffer base to neutralise acid)
• SaO_2 (oxygen saturation)
• HCO_3 or bicarbonate (derived).

Reference ranges:	pH	7.35–7.45
	pCO_2	4.7–6.0 kPa
	pO_2	10.6–13.3 kPa
	Base excess	± 3 mmol/L
	SaO_2	> 94%
	HCO_3	22–30 mmol/L

Specimen:	Whole arterial blood drawn anaerobically into a special heparinised syringe or capilliary tube and transported on ice immediately (within 5–10 minutes) to the laboratory
	Causes for rejection: clotted, inappropriate container, anticoagulant other than sodium or lithium heparin, blood leaking from syringe into ice, large air space or bubbles in syringe, syringe with needle attached.

Causes of low pH (acidosis)	Causes of high pH (alkalosis)

Metabolic acidosis:
  Lactic acidosis
  Diabetic ketoacidosis
  Renal failure
  Renal tubular acidosis
  Severe diarrhoea (loss of bicarbonate)
  Drugs: salicylates
  Ethanol, ethylene glycol or methanol
Respiratory acidosis:
  Lung disease (emphysema, asthma, COPD)
  Neuromuscular (Guillain-Barre syndrome)
  CNS disease (trauma, infection, tumours)
  Drugs: sedatives, anaethetics
	Metabolic alkalosis:
	  Vomiting
	  Hypokalaemia
	  Mineralocorticoid excess (e.g. Cushing's)
	Respiratory alkalosis:
	  Lung disease (pneumonia, asthma, tumours, embolism)
	  Septicaemia (gram –ve)
	  Liver failure
	  Drugs: salicylates
	  Hysterical overbreathing

Calcium

Calcium has a vital role in many physiological and biochemical processes as well as in the structure of bone. Serum calcium is an important determinant of the excitability of nerve and muscle cells.

Approximately 50% of calcium in the blood is bound to proteins (mainly albumin) and about 50% is unbound or ionised. It is the ionised fraction, which is physiologically active. Most laboratories measure total calcium but some report corrected calcium (if albumin is abnormal).

Hypercalcaemia is often discovered incidently. It can cause abdominal pain, constipation, thirst and polyuria.

Hypocalcaemia can cause paraesthesiae, muscle cramps and spasm and rarely convulsions.

Reference range:	2.10–2.60 µmol/L
Sample:	whole blood

Causes of high calcium	Causes of low calcium
Malignancy (with or without metastases) Primary hyperparathyroidism Dehydration (if albumin is increased) Thiazide diuretics (mild) Sarcoidosis Vitamin D intoxication	Vitamin D deficiency (rickets or osteomalacia) Chronic renal failure Hypoparathyroidism

Useful tips

- Abnormal serum albumin concentrations affect total serum calcium. To correct for albumin concentration:
  Corrected calcium = measured calcium + 0.02 x (40 - albumin g/L)
- Acidosis increases ionised calcium and alkalosis decreases ionised calcium. In these situations, patients may show symptoms/signs of hypocalcaemia or hypercalcaemia despite having normal total calcium. In severe acid-base disturbances, ionised calcium should be measured directly.
- Stasis during venepuncture (from tourniquet) may give a falsely raised calcium.

Cholesterol

Cholesterol circulates in the blood incorporated into particles called lipoproteins. The two principal lipoproteins, which contain cholesterol, are low density lipoprotein (LDL) and high density lipoprotein (HDL). High LDL levels are associated with high risk of coronary heart disease (CHD), whereas HDL levels are inversely correlated with CHD (ie. HDL is protective).

High serum cholesterol (due to an excess in LDL) is an important risk factor for atherosclerosis and there is strong evidence that lowering serum cholesterol reduces the risk of CHD and stroke.

Reference ranges should not be used for cholesterol since CHD risk exists within a wide range of concentrations seen in healthy individuals. The desirable cholesterol concentration depends on the presence of other coronary risk factors and whether the patient has existing coronary disease. Generally, the desirable cholesterol concentration is less than 5.0 mmol/L.

Desirable levels:	Total cholesterol <5.0 mmol/L
	LDL cholesterol <3.0 mmol/L
	HDL cholesterol >1.1 mmol/L
Specimen:	whole blood

Causes of high cholesterol	Causes of low cholesterol
Familial Acquired: hypothyroidism, liver disease, renal failure, nephritic syndrome	Acute or chronic illness of any type

Useful tips

- Fasting is not strictly necessary if only total cholesterol is required. Overnight fasting is required if a full lipid profile is required.
- In patients with suspected myocardial infarction (MI), cholesterol should be measured within 24 hours of admission. After 24 hours, and for the following three months, cholesterol may be falsely low.

Cortisol

Cortisol is a hormone secreted by the adrenal gland and is involved in mediating the body's response to stress, maintenance of blood pressure and fluid balance.

Serum cortisol shows a diurnal variation with a peak at 9.00 am and a trough at around midnight. Plasma concentrations are increased by stress from any cause (including surgery and infection).

Reference range (9.00 am):	200–600 nmol/L
Specimen:	whole blood

Causes of high cortisol	Causes of low cortisol
Stress of any cause Cushing's syndrome	Hypoadrenalism

Useful tips

■ There is a wide variation in normal serum cortisol between individuals (see reference range) and therefore measuring a random cortisol is often unhelpful. However, a cortisol below 100 nmol/L is strongly suggestive of hypoadrenalism.
■ Cortisol should not be measured in patients taking steroids since steroids in pharmacological doses will suppress endogenous cortisol production and may also interfere with the cortisol assay.

C-Reactive Protein (CRP)

CRP is a marker of acute inflammation and infection. Its measurement is useful in the management of patients with inflammatory diseases, such as rheumatoid arthritis or Crohn's disease, when it can provide an early indication or an exacerbation (increase) or of response to treatment (decrease).

Reference range:	<5 mg/L
Specimen:	whole blood

Causes of high CRP	Causes of low CRP
Infection (particularly bacterial) Inflammation of any cause	None

Useful tips

■ CRP is a sensitive marker of acute inflammation/infection. It rises within six to 12 hours and peaks at about 48 hours following the onset of inflammation/infection.
■ Very high CRP concentrations are usually associated with bacterial infection.
■ CRP can be suppressed by salicylates, steroids, or non-steroidal anti-inflammatory agents.

Creatine kinase (CK)

CK is an enzyme, which is present in high concentration in skeletal (CK-MM isoenzyme) and cardiac muscle (CK-MB isoenzyme). Its major use is in the diagnosis and management of muscle disease. Its use in the investigation of chest pain has now been superseded by cardiac troponins (see below).

Reference range:	<170 IU/L
Specimen:	whole blood

Causes of high CK	Causes of low CK
Myopathy and muscular dystrophies Muscle injury (trauma, surgery, exercise) Myositis (viral, alcholic) Myocardial damage (MI, cardioversion) Central nervous system: stroke, meningitis, head injury Pulmonary or intestinal infarction Others: hypothyroidism, sepsis, shock and acute psychosis	None

Useful tips

- CK activity may be raised immediately after exercise and it reaches a peak after one to two days. The more severe the exercise, the higher the increase in CK. The effect on CK is more pronounced in subjects who do not exercise regularly.
- Afro-Caribbeans (particularly males) have up to twice the CK level found in Caucasians. Asians have intermediate values.

Creatinine

Creatinine is a waste product of muscle metabolism. It is produced at a constant rate and is excreted in the urine. Its measurement in serum is used as a test of renal function but the glomerular filtration rate (GFR) must fall to about half the normal before serum creatinine is increased.

Reference range (adult):	60–120 µmol/L
Specimen:	whole blood

Causes of high creatinine	Causes of low creatinine
Renal failure (acute or chronic)	Children Severe muscle wasting

Useful tips

- In early renal disease, serum creatinine may be within the reference range despite a reduced GFR.
- When interpreting serum creatinine, muscle mass must be taken into account.
- A recent meal including meat, particularly if stewed, may cause a transient increase in serum creatinine concentration.

Gamma-glutamyltransferase (GGT)

GGT is an enzyme which is mainly present in the liver. High GGT can occur in all types of liver disease but it is particularly useful as an indicator of excessive alcohol consumption.

Reference range:	<58 IU/L
Speciment:	whole blood

Causes of high GGT	Causes of low GGT
Hepatitis Cholestatic liver disease Excessive alcohol consumption Drugs: anticonvulsants, amitriptyline, warfarin Fatty liver (diabetes mellitus, obesity)	None

Useful tips

- If the origin of a raised ALP is uncertain, a concomitant elevation of GGT will suggest that the raised ALP is of hepatic origin.

- The half-life of serum GGT is about 26 days and, consequently, in patients with very high initial GGT activities, due to excessive alcohol intake, elevated levels can be found even after an abstinence period of longer than one month.

Glucose

In healthy subjects, the blood glucose concentration is maintained within relatively narrow limits through a tightly controlled balance between glucose production and glucose utilisation. After an overnight fast, blood glucose is usually between 4.5–5.2 mmol/L. After meals, glucose levels increase but typical meals will not raise glucose above 10.0 mmol/L, and normal levels are usually restored within two to four hours.

In stress, due to injury or infection, the concentrations of various hormones (catecholamines, cortisol, glucagons and growth hormone) increase causing insulin resistance and consequently raised blood glucose levels.

Reference range (fasting):	4.5–5.2 mmol/L
Specimen (fluoride oxalate):	whole blood

Causes of high blood glucose	Causes of low blood glucose
Diabetes mellitus Impaired glucose tolerance Severe stress	Tumours: insulinoma, non-islet cell tumours Endocrine deficiencies: Addison's disease, hypopituitarism Drugs: insulin, sulphonylureas, quinine, salicylates, beta-blockers Autoimmune hypoglycaemia (rare)

Useful tips

- Diabetes mellitus can be diagnosed if fasting plasma glucose is ≥7.0 mmol/L or random glucose >11.0 mmol/L in a patient with symptoms of diabetes, or on more than one occasion in a patient without symptoms.
- Diabetes should never be diagnosed on the basis of glycosuria alone.
- A random glucose result can only be interpreted in relation to the time of the previous meal. If random glucose is 5.5–11.0 mmol/L, measurement should be repeated after fasting.

Phosphate

Phosphate is usually measured with calcium and alkaline phosphatase as part of a 'bone profile'. It is an essential precursor of high-energy phosphate compounds (eg ATP) and a component of nucleic acids, phospholipids and bone. Severe hypophosphataemia can cause muscle weakness.

Reference range (adult):	0.8–1.4 mmol/L
Specimen:	whole blood

Causes of high phosphate	Causes of low phosphate
Renal failure Bone tumours (especially metastatic)	Starvation or malnutrition Dextrose infusions Alcohol withdrawal Hyperparathyroidism Renal tubular disease

Useful tips

- Serum phosphate usually increases after meals.
- Haemolysis gives falsely raised values.

Potassium

Potassium is the major intracellular cation but its plasma concentration has a major effect on the excitability of nerve and muscle membranes. It is measured as part of the 'renal profile'.

Hypokalaemia causes muscle weakness, cardiac dysrhythmias, constipation, thirst, polyuria and intestinal pseudo-obstruction.

Hyperkalaemia is often clinically silent, but at concentrations of >6.5 mmol/L there is an increased risk of cardiac arrest.

Reference range:	3.8–5.2 mmol/L
Specimen:	whole blood, freshly drawn

Causes of hyperkalaemia	Causes of hypokalaemia
Renal failure	Gastrointestinal loss: diarrhoea, laxatives
Potassium-sparing diuretics	Renal loss: thiazides and loop diuretics
Acidosis (except Renal Tubular Acidosis)	Dextrose infusions
Addison's disease	Alkalosis of any cause
Hypoaldosteronism	Cushing's syndrome
Pseudo-hyperkalaemia: Haemolysis, delay in separation of cells from serum	Primary hyperaldosteronism

Useful tips

- Haemolysis and delay in separation of cells from serum can cause falsely high results or can cause genuinely low potassium levels to appear normal.
- Serum potassium is usually higher than plasma potassium. Therefore, borderline raised serum potassium should be repeated in a lithium heparin bottle (plasma potassium).

Sodium

Sodium is the major extracellular cation and its plasma concentration is the determinant of extracellular fluid osmolality and volume. Sodium is usually measured as part of a 'renal profile' and its abnormalities can be related to abnormal water or sodium homeostasis.

Hyponatraemia is relatively common in hospitalised patients but is often mild and asymptomatic. When severe (<120 mmol/L), it may cause confusion, disorientation, ataxia and coma.

Hypernatraemia is less common and is usually due to dehydration.

Reference range:	135–145 mmol/L
Specimen:	whole blood

Causes of hypernatraemia	Causes of hyponatraemia

Dehydration
Diabetes insipidus
Excessive salt intake (oral or
  parenteral)
Spurious: contamination (eg blood
  collected from an arm with an
  intravenous infusion running)
	Salt loss:
	  Gastrointestinal (diarrhoea & vomiting)
	  Renal (diuretics, adrenal failure)
	  Skin (burns)
	Water overload:
	  Oedematous states (cirrhosis, CCF)
	  Renal failure (acute or chronic)
	  Inappropriate IV fluid regime
	  Psychogenic polydipsia
	  Syndrome of Inappropriate Anti-Diuretic Hormone (SIADH)
	Spurious: contamination (eg blood collected from an arm
	  with an intravenous infusion running)

Useful tips

- Blood should never be collected from an arm with an intravenous infusion running, as this can give erroneous results and may therefore result in inappropriate treatment.
- Mild hyponatraemia is relatively common in hospitalised patients and does not usually require further investigation.
- If hyponatraemia is severe (serum sodium <120 mmol/L), serum and urine osmolalities should be measured and clinical assessment should be made.
- Clinical signs are useful in indicating whether hyponatraemia is due to salt loss or water overload. Thirst and low blood pressure (BP) would suggest salt loss, whereas a normal/high BP would suggest water overload.
- In patients with hyponatraemia, a high serum urea concentration would suggest salt loss, whereas a low serum urea would suggest water overload (eg SIADH).

Thyroid Function tests (TFT)

The thyroid gland produces thyroxine (T4) and tri-iodothyronine (T3). This production is regulated by thyrotropin or thyroid-stimulating hormone (TSH) produced by the pituitary gland. T4 and T3 are extensively protein bound in the plasma but only the free hormones are physiologically active. Most laboratories nowadays measure the free hormone concentrations (FT4 and FT3) in addition to TSH.

Many laboratories measure serum TSH as a first line test and other tests (FT4, FT3 or both) are only added if TSH is abnormal. In **primary hypothyroidism**, the TSH is typically high and FT4 is low. In mild or early disease, TSH may be elevated but FT4 may be normal or low-normal. In

secondary hypothyroidism (secondary to pituitary failure), FT4 is low and TSH is also low or inappropriately normal. In **hyperthyroidism**, TSH is suppressed and both FT4 and FT3 are high.

Reference ranges:	TSH	0.4–4.0 mIU/L
	FT4	10.6–21.0 pmol/L
	FT3	3.2–5.9 pmol/L
Reference ranges may vary between laboratories		
Specimen:	whole blood	

Useful tips

- **Sick euthyroid syndrome** In hospitalised patients, thyroid function tests can often be misleading. Therefore, TFT should not be requested on hospitalised patients unless the main presenting feature is thought to be related to a thyroid disorder (eg. atrial fibrillation, hypothermia).
- **Drugs and thyroid function** A number of medications are well known to affect thyroid function. Glucocorticoids and dopamine can lower the serum TSH level; lithium may cause hypothyroidism in 5 - 10% of patients; iodide, as used in iodine-containing sterilising solution, radio-opaque dyes or amiodarone, can cause hyperthyroidism in predisposed individuals; amiodarone can itself directly cause hyper- or hypothyroidism by a direct effect on the thyroid gland.

Troponins: cardiac Troponin I (cTnI) and T (cTnT)

Troponins (I, T and C) are components of the muscle contractile structure. Assays have been developed for the detection of cardiac-specific forms of troponin: cardiac Troponin I (cTnI) and cardiac Troponin T (cTnT). These assays are sensitive and specific markers of myocardial injury.

After the onset of acute myocardial infarction (AMI), blood levels of troponins start to rise at four to six hours and peak at about 18-24 hours. They remain elevated in the serum for six to ten days.

Reference ranges (cTnI):	<0.1 ng/ml	Negative
	0.1–0.25 ng/ml	Intermediate
	>0.25 ng/ml	Positive
Specimen:	whole blood	

Causes of high troponin
Acute myocardial Infarction (AMI)
Myocarditis
Congestive cardiac failure
Unstable angina
Chest trauma
Cardiac surgery

Useful tips:

- Troponins are not 'early markers' of cardiac damage. A negative value on blood collected less than 12 hours after onset of chest pain does not exclude cardiac damage.
- Troponins (cTnI and cTnT) do not rise with skeletal muscle damage.
- Elevated levels of troponins can be found in patients with chronic renal failure including those on dialysis treatment.
- False positive results may be due to interference from antibodies in the patient serum. Therefore, troponin results must be taken in context with the patient's clinical circumstances.

Tumour markers

Tumour markers are substances secreted into body fluids or expressed on cell surfaces, which are characteristic of the presence of a tumour. Generally, tumour markers are of potential value in the diagnosis, prognosis and in assessing the response to treatment. In practice, however, the number of tumour markers of proven value in the management of malignancy is small. The commonly performed tumour markers are alpha-fetoprotein (AFP), Ovarian marker (CA 125), carcino-embryonic antigen (CEA), human chorionic gonadotrophin (HCG) and prostate specific antigen (PSA).

General points

- No serum marker in current use is specific for malignancy.
- Generally, serum marker levels are rarely elevated in patients with early malignancy.
- Very few markers have absolute organ specificity.
- Most tumour markers do not have sufficient sensitivity or specificity to make their measurements reliable in the diagnosis or exclusion of cancer.
- Requesting of multiple markers (AFP, CEA, HCG and CA 125) in an attempt to identify an unknown primary cancer is rarely of use.

Urea

Urea is the major end product of protein metabolism. It is synthesised in the liver and excreted by the kidneys. It is often measured as part of the 'renal profile' ie urea and electrolytes or U&E's, but creatinine (see above) provides a better index of renal function.

Reference range:	2.5–6.5 mmol/L
Specimen:	whole blood

Causes of high urea	Causes of low urea
Renal failure Dehydration High protein intake Gastrointestinal bleeding (due to catabolism of retained blood)	Starvation

Uric acid

Uric acid (urate) is the end product of nucleic acid metabolism (cell nuclei). Uric acid is excreted in urine and increases in serum uric acid may be caused by either increased production or decreased excretion. High uric acid concentrations can predispose to gout, due to deposition of urate crystals in joints.

Reference range (men):	200–500 µmol/L
(women):	200–400 µmol/L
Specimen:	whole blood

Causes of high uric acid	Causes of low uric acid
Renal failure Gout Cancer Pre-eclampsia Starvation Diabetic ketoacidosis Trauma Drugs: thiazide diuretics	Hypouricaemia is uncommon and is of no clinical consequence

Urinalysis

Dipstick testing of urine is useful in screening for certain disorders and in pointing the way to further investigations. Tests for protein, pH, blood, leucocytes, glucose, bilirubin, urobilinogen, ketones and specific gravity are available. The number of tests on each stick depends on the brand and type used.

Bilirubin

- A positive test indicates an elevation of conjugated bilirubin in the plasma which is indicative of hepatobiliary disease.
- A positive test may precede clinical jaundice.

Blood

- The presence of blood in urine should always be further investigated (provided that contamination, e.g. with menstrual bleeding, can be excluded).
- A positive test may indicate haematuria or myoglobinuria and therefore should be sent to Microbiology for microscopic examination.
- Causes of a positive test include renal disease, urinary tract infection or tumours, renal stones and rhabdomyolysis (muscle breakdown).

Glucose

- Glycosuria indicates either diabetes or a low renal threshold for glucose.
- A positive test in a non-diabetic patient should always be followed by measurement of blood glucose.
- The diagnosis of diabetes should never be made solely on the finding of a positive urine dipstick.

pH

- Knowledge of urine pH is rarely of diagnostic value.
- A high urine pH (>7.5) may result in falsely low result for protein.

Ketones

- Testing for ketones is useful in patients with diabetes mellitus, as ketonuria in a patient with type 1 diabetes (insulin-dependent) suggests a developing ketoacidosis.
- Ketonuria can also occur in non-diabetic patients who are losing weight.

Leucocytes

- The test is useful as a screening test for urinary tract infection.
- A positive test should be followed by urine microscopy and culture.

Protein

- The test detects albumin at concentrations as low as 200 mg/L.
- Proteinuria can occur in renal disease, urinary tract infections or can be an incidental finding.
- A positive test should always be followed up.

Urobilinogen

- The presence or absence of urobilinogen is of little diagnostic significance.

Haematology

Full blood count

Laboratories rely on automated counters to provide information on haemoglobin concentration (Hb), red blood cell count (RBC), mean corpuscular volume (MCV) and white blood cell count (WBC). Other red cell indices such as packed cell volume (PCV), mean corpuscular haemoglobin (MCH) and mean corpuscular haemoglobin concentration (MCHC) are derived.

Automated counters recognise leucocytes as nucleated cells and differentials (neutrophils, lymphocytes, monocytes and eosinophils) are obtained on the basis of relative nuclear size to the cell, nuclear complexity, and the presence of cytoplasmic granules.

Reference ranges:	Men	Women	(Unit)
Hb	14.0–18.0	12.0–16.0	(g/dL)
RBC	4.5–6.0	4.2–5.4	$(x\ 10^{12}/L)$
WCC	4.0–11.0	4.0–11.0	$(x\ 10^{9}/L)$
Platelets	150–400	150–400	$(x\ 10^{9}/L)$
Specimen:	whole blood		
Reference ranges depend on age and sex			

Haemoglobin (Hb) and red blood cells (RBC)

Red blood cells are highly specialised cells, which are filled with haemoglobin, and have a life span of approximately 120 days.

Haemoglobin is a unique oxygen-binding molecule for the efficient uptake of oxygen in the high partial pressure environment of the lungs, avidly retaining it while circulating in the arterial vasculature and releasing it when the appropriate pressures are reached in the capillary bed.

Anaemia, a decrease in the number of red cells, can be due to decreased red cell production, increased destruction or blood loss. Polycythaemia, an increase in circulating red blood cells, can be due to an increase in red cell mass or to a decrease in plasma volume.

Causes of low Hb and RBC	Causes of high Hb and RBC
Anaemia of any cause	Polycythaemia
Iron, vitamin B12 or folate deficiency	Haemoconcentration (dehydration)
Haemodilution (eg excessive IV fluids, pregnancy)	Chronic obstructive pulmonary disease (COPD)
Haemorrhage	Smoking
Haemolysis	Pre-eclampsia
Chronic renal failure	
Chronic liver disease	

Useful tips

- Smokers typically have elevated haemoglobin levels in response to chronic, low grade carbon monoxide poisoning and other respiratory ailments. Because of the carbon monoxide binding, these patients may still be functionally anaemic even though their haemoglobin levels appear higher than normal.
- During the initial phase of acute haemorrhage, haemoglobin levels do not change very much. After several hours, as extracellular fluid is mobilised and intravenous fluids are given, haemoglobin levels go down due to the dilutional effects.

White blood cells (WBC)

White blood cells are produced in the bone marrow, lymph nodes, the spleen and thymus. They fight infection and foreign bodies and help distribute antibodies throughout the body. Unused, a white blood cell lives for two to three weeks, and then disintegrates.

Causes of high WBC	Causes of low WBC

Infection
Haemorrhage
Trauma
Some malignancies
Exposure to toxic substances
Renal failure
Drugs: e.g. quinine, adrenaline
Chronic inflammatory conditions
Stress reaction
Exercise, heat and cold
Anaesthesia
Smoking
	Viral infections
	Bone marrow depression, secondary to:
	    Drugs: analgesics, antibiotics, antihistaminics,
	    anticonvulsants, anti-inflammatory drugs,
	    antithyroid drugs, barbiturates, chemotherapy
	    and diuretics
	Arsenic and heavy metal exposure
	Radiation exposure

Platelets

Platelets are formed primarily in the bone marrow. They are released into the blood stream where they normally live for about a week. Platelets serve to assist in clotting, coagulation and in maintaining vascular integrity.

Causes of increased platelets (thrombocytosis)	Causes of decreased platelets (thrombocytopenia)
Infection Infections Inflammation or trauma Cancer Bleeding Athletes and high altitudes	Haemorrhage Infections Liver disease Disseminated intravascular coagulopathy (DIC) Severe pre-eclampsia HELLP syndrome (Haemolysis, Elevated Liver enzymes, Low Platelets) Allergic reactions Drugs: NSAID, diuretics Alcohol excess Bone marrow suppression Idiopathic thrombocytopenic purpura (ITP)

Useful tips

- Abnormal bleeding due to low platelet counts does not normally occur until platelets fall below 50×10^9/L.
- Aspirin affects platelet function causing abnormal bleeding despite a normal platelet count.
- After discontinuation of aspirin, platelet function will be regained within 7 days.
- Platelet count may be falsely low because of 'clumping'.

Erythrocyte sedimentation rate (ESR)

The ESR is the speed at which non-clotted red blood cells settle to the bottom of a test tube. Increased rates of RBC settling are caused by changes in plasma proteins following tissue damage or during inflammation.

Reference ranges:	Men	Women
	0–5 mm/hr	0–7 mm/hr
Specimen:	whole blood (EDTA or citrated)	

Causes of high ESR
Inflammation or infection (due to increase in plasma proteins) Chronic disease (due to increase in immunoglobin) Pregnancy (due to raised fibrinogen) Elderly (due to reduced plasma albumin)

Coagulation screen

The coagulation screen is usually requested on patients with bleeding or who bruise easily. The coagulation screen includes **prothrombin time (PT)** and **activated partial thromboplastin time (APTT or PTTK)**.

Reference ranges:	PT	10–13 seconds
	APTT (PTTK)	25–35 seconds
Specimen:	whole blood (citrated)	

Prothrombin time (PT):

PT is a measure of how long it takes the blood to clot. At least a dozen blood-clotting factors are needed for blood to clot normally. PT is an important coagulation test because it measures the presence and activity of five different vitamin K dependent clotting factors (factors I, II, V, VII and X).

Causes of prolonged PT
Liver disease
Vitamin K deficiency (secondary to malabsorption)
Warfarin therapy
Factor I, II, V, VII or X deficiency

Activated partial thromboplastin time (APTT):

APTT (PTTK) is a functional measure of the intrinsic pathway of coagulation activation.

Causes of prolonged APPT
Liver disease
Deficiency of one or more of the clotting factors
Presence of inhibitors e.g. Lupus anticoagulant (in systemic lupus erythematosis, neoplasia)
Heparin therapy

International normalised ratio (INR)

Because normal values may vary from one laboratory to another, a method of standardising prothrombin time results, called the **international normalised ratio (INR)** has been used. The INR is a prothrombin time ratio (normal/control), which has been corrected for the type of thromboplastin used. This method of expression ensures that INR results are equivalent both over time and between laboratories.

The INR is used in patients on anticoagulant therapy (warfarin), in the majority of whom the INR is usually kept between 2 and 3 to prevent blood clots from forming. For patients with mechanical prosthetic heart valves or recurrent thromembolic disease, a higher INR of 3–4.5 is recommended.

Blood transfusion

Where possible, patients who are likely to need a blood transfusion should receive the National Blood Service leaflet Receiving a Blood Transfusion; A leaflet for patients and their relatives'.

Obtaining blood specimens for cross-match (X-match):

- The blood specimen should be obtained using the approved procedure.
- Blood should be collected into a plain X-match bottle.
- Patient details should be hand-written on the X-match form and all questions on the form must be answered.
- All details should be checked with the patient's notes, patient's wristband and, if possible, confirmed by the patient.
- The specimen should be labelled with the patient's name, unit number, date of birth and address.
- The specimen should be dated, timed and signed immediately after collection.
- Blood should not be collected from an arm with an IV infusion in-situ.
- All high-risk specimens must have self-adhesive Biohazard labels attached and be packed in a sealable plastic specimen bag.

Collecting blood products from the blood bank fridge:

- When blood or platelet bags are removed from the blood bank, the person removing the bags should check the patient's details from the prescription sheet/patient's notes against the bag removed and must sign, date and time the laboratory copy, which is kept in the blood bank. The white form should be filled after the transfusion has been completed and should be kept in patient's notes.
- Units of blood or platelets must be taken and used in the order stated on the form.
- Only one unit of blood per patient should normally be removed from the blood bank fridge at any one time. In cases of massive blood loss, where more units are needed, they should be transported in an appropriate container, which will be supplied by the blood bank on request.
- Transport boxes are only suitable for storage of blood for a maximum of two hours.
- Unused units must be returned to the issue fridge as soon as possible with the time of return documented on the blue copy of the X-match form.
- The total transfusion episode, from signing out of the issue fridge to completion of the transfusion must be within five hours.
- If the decision to transfuse is cancelled and the blood is returned within 30 minutes of removal, record the date and time of return on the blue copy of the X-match form. If the unit has been out of the issue fridge for 30 minutes or longer, do not return to the issue fridge. Contact blood bank staff for advice.

Microbiology

- Specimens for microbiological tests must be transported in robust and leak-proof containers.
- Specimens must be placed individually in self-sealing plastic bags.
- Specimens from patients suspected of having hepatitis B or HIV infection must be securely packaged and the request form and specimen should bear 'Danger of Infection' labels.

Urine culture and sensitivity

Urine is normally sterile. However, in the process of collecting the urine, some contamination from skin bacteria is frequent. For that reason, up to 10,000 colonies of bacteria/mL are considered normal and only greater than 100,000 colonies/mL represents urinary tract infection.

Before a 'mid-stream' urine sample is taken, the urethral meatus should be carefully cleaned with soap and water or a wipe. In catheterised patients, samples should be aspirated from the tubing, not taken from the collection bag. A report stating 'heavy mixed growth' means that two or more types of organisms have been cultured; as true mixed infections are extremely rare, it is likely that either the culture was contaminated when taken, or there was a delay in culture which led to overgrowth of some organisms.

Sensitivity refers to the antibiotics tested to be effective in stopping the bacteria. While clinical response will generally follow therapy guided by sensitivity testing, the response can be variable.

Indications for urine microscopy, culture and sensitivity

- cystitis
- pyelonephritis
- prostatitis
- suspected urinary tract infection in children
- assessment of unwell patients who are permanently catheterised
- suspected tuberculosis (TB)
- immuno-compromised patients
- pregnancy (on booking/first presentation).

Throat culture

Throat culture may be obtained for nearly any microorganism, but is usually performed to detect streptococcal infection. The throat swab must be taken with reasonable pressure against the fauces and tonsils and placed in a tube of transport medium.

Indications for a throat swab

- severe sore throat

- acute cervical lymphadenopathy
- oral ulceration (herpetic, gingivitis)
- screening for carriage of methicillin-resistant staphylococcus aureus (MRSA).

Blood culture

Particular care must be taken to avoid skin bacterial contamination when blood cultures are drawn. The skin should be cleaned for 30 seconds with isopropyl alcohol and allowed to dry. After the blood is drawn, the needle should be replaced with a fresh sterile needle before injecting the blood into the culture bottle.

Indications for blood culture

- high fevers or rigors
- fever of unknown origin
- immunocompromised patients or indwelling Hickman line
- diabetic patients with cellulitis or infected foot ulcer
- pneumonia especially post-influenzal
- abdominal sepsis
- pyelonephritis.

Stool culture

Stool normally has a large number of various organisms present. Stool should be passed directly into a collection jar or a bedpan. A sample can be separated with a tongue blade and placed into a specimen container.

Stool cultures are used to identify viruses, parasites and other pathogenic micro-organisms. The routine culture can identify shigella, salmonella, campylobacter, and E. Coli 0157.

Indications for stool microscopy and culture

- significant diarrhoea of any cause
- diarrhoea in a patient who has returned from abroad in the previous month
- diarrhoea in immunocompromised patients

- diarrhoea with significant systemic symptoms.

Cerebrospinal fluid (CSF)

CSF is normally sterile, colourless and clear. It contains most of the same constituents as blood, but generally in lower concentrations.

In bacterial meningitis CSF is cloudy, WBCs are primarily neutrophils and CSF glucose is generally decreased. In non-bacterial meningitis CSF is clear and CSF glucose is normal or decreased.

Causes of yellow CSF:

- previous subarachnoid bleeding
- severe jaundice
- high concentrations of protein (>1.5 g/L).

Causes of bloody CSF:

- bloody tap
- subarachnoid or cerebral haemorrhage
- at least 400 RBC/ml must be present before CSF is visibly bloody.

Causes of cloudy CSF:

- infection (bacterial or other microorganisms)
- increased WBC or RBC count.

Hepatitis serology

Hepatitis serology for hepatitis A, B and C is indicated in all patients with jaundice and in certain high risk patients.

Hepatitis A

- is transmitted by the faecal/oral route
- affects children and young adults more often
- is not associated with chronic hepatitis or a carrier status
- has an incubation period of two to six weeks
- hepatitis A IgM will be elevated from six to 14 weeks after infection.

Hepatitis B

- is transmitted parenterally (drug injection or blood transfusion)
- 10% of patients become carriers
- has an incubation period of six to 26 weeks
- hepatitis B surface antigen (HbsAg) appears in the serum four to 12 weeks following infection
- hepatitis B core antibody appears within six to 14 weeks
- hepatitis B surface antibody appears four to ten months following infection, indicating clinical recovery and immunity to the virus.

Hepatitis C

- is transmitted parenterally (drug injection, needlestick injury or blood transfusion)
- 80% of persons have no signs or symptoms
- is associated with high rates of chronic hepatitis with progression to cirrhosis
- persons at risk of hepatitis C might also be at risk for infection with hepatitis B virus or HIV.

Human immunodeficiency virus (HIV)

- is carried in certain body fluids including blood, semen, vaginal secretions and breast milk
- is transmitted through sexual contact, needlestick injury, during birth or breast-feeding
- HIV infects and destroys white blood cells called CD4+T, which are cells of the immune system that protect against infections

- acquired immune deficiency syndrome (AIDS) develops when the body succumbs to opportunistic infections or cancers that take advantage of the body's lowered defences
- HIV antibodies generally appear within three months after infection with HIV, but may take up to six months in some patients.

Methicillin-resistant staphylococcus aureus (MRSA)

- Staphylococcus aureus, often referred to simply as 'staph', are bacteria commonly carried in the skin or in the nose of healthy people.
- Occasionally, staph can cause infections but most of these are minor (eg boils) and most can be treated with antibiotics. However, staph can cause serious infections, such as surgical wound infections and pneumonia.
- Over the past 50 years, treatment of staph infections has become more difficult because staph bacteria have become resistant to various antibiotics, including the commonly used penicillin-related antibiotics. These resistant bacteria are called MRSA.
- MRSA infection occurs more commonly among persons in hospitals and healthcare facilities. It usually develops in hospitalised patients who are elderly or very sick or who have an open wound (eg. bedsore) or a tube (eg urinary catheter or I.V. catheter).
- MRSA can spread among people having close contact with infected people. It is almost always spread by direct physical contact, and not through the air. Spread may also occur indirectly by touching objects (eg. towels, sheets, wound dressings) contaminated by the infected skin.

Screening patients or staff for MRSA carriage

- **When**: Staff should be screened before starting work and patients on admission/pre-admission to hospital, if they have been in a healthcare facility in the previous six months, where cross-transmission may have occurred. Screening may also occur as part of an outbreak investigation in conjunction with the infection control officer.
- **How**: One nasal swab (both anterior nares), one swab from the perineum and swabs from any skin lesions, surgical wounds or catheter sites.

Clostridium difficile (C. difficile)

- C. difficile is carried as part of the normal gut flora in very young children.
- In adults, particularly those who are elderly or very sick who have previously received antibiotics, it can cause a severe diarrhoeal illness.
- C. difficile can be spread by direct physical contact and also by contact with contaminated hospital equipment (eg commodes).

Remember:

- To check with your local laboratory
  - When result do not seem appropriate
  - For reference ranges

Additional reading

Malarkey L, McMorrow ME, and Eoyang T (eds) (2000) Nurse's Manual of Laboratory Tests and Diagnostic Procedures (second edition). WB Saunders, Philadelphia

Fischbach FT (ed) (1997) Common Laboratory and Diagnostic Tests (second edition). WB Saunders, Philadelphia

Helpful websites

www.blood.co.uk
www.labtestsonline.org
www.rcpamanual.edu.au

Chapter 9

Medicines management

Ann Close

The safe storage, custody and administration of medicines are an integral part of the nurse's role and increasingly nurses are becoming involved in prescribing. Medicines also form a key part of many patients' treatment. However, medication errors are a persistent problem. Mostly these relate to prescribing and administration of medicines but problems with the safe storage and custody arise from time to time

This chapter will look at the role of the nurse in safe storage of medicines, good practice in administration and factors which contribute to errors and the actions that can be taken to minimise risks.

Legal and professional documentation

There are a number of legal and professional documents which provide a framework for the safe storage, custody and administration of medicines.

1. The Medicines Act 1968

This together with subsequent Statutory Instruments provides the legal framework for the manufacture, licensing, prescription, supply and administration of medicines. It classifies medicines into:

- prescription only medicines – those supplied or administered to a patient on the instruction of an appropriate practitioner
- pharmacy only medicines – those purchased from a pharmacy under the supervision of a pharmacist
- general sale list – those that can be obtained from retail outlets and do not need a prescription or to be sold under the supervision of a pharmacist.

2. Misuse of Drugs Act 1971

This legislation is concerned with controlled drugs and categorises them into five schedules. Schedule 2 and 3 are relevant to nursing:

- schedule 2 medicines eg. morphine, diamorphine and pethidine
- schedule 3 medicines eg. barbiturates.

3. The Nursing and Midwifery Council

Guidelines for the administration of medicines (NMC, 2004). This sets out the standards expected of registered nurses in relation to medicines management.

4. Review of prescribing, supply and administration of medicines (The Crown Report)

In 1997 a team led by Dr June Crown was established to undertake a review of prescribing, supply and administration of medicines. In 1998 an interim report was produced about the supply and administration of medicines by nurses under group protocols as the legal position was uncertain at the time.

Patient Group Direction is a specific written instruction for the supply or administration of named medicines in an identified clinical situation. It is drawn up locally by doctors, pharmacists and other appropriate professionals and approved by the employer, advised by the relevant professional advisory committees. It applies to groups of patients or other service users who may not be individually identified before the presentation for treatment.' (Crown report 1998).

The final report was produced in 1999 which has provided nurses with the opportunity to develop as:

Independent prescribers are professionals who are responsible for the initial assessment of the patient and for devising the broad treatment plan with the authority to prescribe the medicines required as part of that plan.

Supplementary prescribers are professionals who are authorised to prescribe certain medicines for patients whose condition has been diagnosed or assessed by an independent prescriber within an agreed assessment and treatment plan.

You should have policies on these in your own organisation.

5. The Clinical Negligence Scheme for Trusts (CNST) risk management standards

CNST have added a new standard from April 2004 on safe medicines practice to ensure that trusts have put into place safeguards which will result in a reduction in the number and cost of claims for medication errors. The standards include the need for induction programmes and continuing professional development on medicines management, the need for risk assessment and adverse incident reporting, policies that will ensure the prescribing, supply, administration and safe custody of medicines comply with legislation and audit of prescription sheets. (NHSLA and Willis, 2003)

6. Your organisation's policy on medicines management and related procedures.

Although it is important for you to have an understanding of the content of the above documents, the essential messages will be incorporated into your organisation's policy and procedure and you should have detailed knowledge of this. Such policies often have additional requirements that take account of the local situation.

Storage and security of medicines within the hospital environment

The ward or department nurse manager has overall responsibility for the safe storage and custody of medicines but in their absence the nurse in charge of the shift acts on their behalf. You should therefore understand your role and responsibilities as a registered nurse in your own area for:

Obtaining medicines

You should ensure:

- Medicines are only obtained via the pharmacy on a signed written order which may be:

- the in-patient treatment chart
- outpatient prescription
- TTO prescription (medicines to take home)

} signed by a doctor or other prescriber

- stock or controlled drug requisition – signed by a registered nurse.
- Blank prescriptions are kept in a locked cupboard or drawer when not in use to prevent unauthorised access.
- Loss or theft of prescriptions and/or requisition order forms are reported to the chief pharmacist and senior nurse.
- Transport of medicines and requisition books is in tamper evident containers or by an authorised person.

Security of the medicine cupboard keys

You should know:

- Who the keys may be passed on to and what should be done with them if the ward temporarily closes, for example, overnight, for the weekend or for refurbishment.
- What should be done if the keys go missing and to whom you should report this.

Storage arrangements in your area

You should know the storage arrangements for:

- Products for internal use.
- IV fluids, irrigation fluids and parenteral use.
- Controlled drugs.
- The medicines trolley.
- The medicines refrigerator.
- Drugs for external use.
- Clinical reagents.
- Emergency drugs for cardiac arrest.

Normally most of the above should be kept in a lockable medicines cupboard when not in use. There are sometimes exceptions and you should be aware of these for your area, for example:

- Emergency medicines kits eg cardiac arrest boxes.
- ITU and theatre medicines cupboards – storing medicines for injections.

Storage of these, however, must be done in such a way as to prevent unauthorised access.

Disposal of medicines

You should be aware of the procedures for the following:

- Returning out of date or stock items no longer required. This is usually to be returned to pharmacy in a locked box.
- Controlled drugs. This is usually done by a pharmacist.
- Disposing of patients' own medicines.

Monitoring stocks

Frequent checks should be made on the stock of medicines held by the ward or department. There are often special instructions for checking controlled drugs and you should be aware of what these are for your area. You should also know the action to take and whom to inform when stocks, prescriptions or requisition books go missing.

Controlled drugs

There are special arrangements for the ordering, transport and receipt of controlled drugs and you should check the specific requirements for your organisation.

- Ordering should be done by a registered nurse.
- Controlled drugs should be transported inside a locked controlled drug box by the relevant messenger service.
- Receiving and checking of controlled drugs should be done by a registered nurse.
- Drugs should be stored in a controlled drugs cupboard - a locked cupboard within a locked cupboard, used solely for that purpose. The registered nurse in charge of the ward is responsible for holding the keys.
- Records of stocks and use of controlled drugs should be kept in the controlled drugs register. Many hospitals require that these are checked at least weekly.
- The patient's own controlled drugs brought into hospital should be returned home immediately if possible. If they cannot be returned home

then they should be kept with the patient's other medication in a sealed bag and stored in a secure manner until the patient is discharged.
- Ampoules which are found broken or are accidentally broken should be reported to the senior nurse.

Medication errors

These include giving the wrong dose or wrong drug, giving medication at the wrong time or by the wrong route or omitting the prescribed drug altogether.

It is important that a 'no blame' culture exists to encourage reporting of medication errors and incidents so that action can be taken to prevent a repeat of the situation. However if an error occurs the following action should be taken:

- The hospital's adverse incident procedure should be followed.
- The patient's doctor should be informed to ensure that action is taken to safeguard the patient's wellbeing.
- The line manager and/or senior nurse should be notified.
- An investigation should be undertaken to find out why the error occurred, this should include an assessment of the context and any contributory factors.
- an action plan should be developed based on the findings of the investigation.

Factors contributing to drug errors

1. The ability of the nurse to calculate doses or administration rates. This is often due to poor mathematical skills (Table 9.1).
2. Nurses knowledge of medication. New medicines are constantly being introduced into the health service that makes it difficult for nurses to keep up to date.
3. Experience and competence of the nurse. Although it could be expected that nurses with more experience are more competent in medicines administration, this has not been demonstrated in research studies (O'Shea, 1999).
4. Working patterns, workload and staffing levels. When staffing levels are poor, the work load increases and there may be frequent interruptions, loss of concentration and shortcuts taken which lead to

mistakes being made.
5. Drug administration policies and procedures. Each organisation has its own medicine management policy and procedure. Where these are complex, long or difficult to follow, there may be insufficient time to read them or a lack of understanding and mistakes will be more likely.

Minimising errors

The NMC (Nursing and Midwifery Council) indicates the following good practice which will help to minimise errors (2004):

- know the therapeutic uses of the medicines to be administered, normal dose, side effects, precautions and contra-indications
- be certain of the identity of the patient
- be aware of patient's care plan
- check the prescription and the label of the dispensed medicine is clearly written and unambiguous
- consider the dosage, method of administration, route and timing of the administration in the context of the condition of the patient and co-existing therapies
- check the expiry date
- check the patient is not allergic to the medicine before it is administered
- contact the prescriber where contra-indications are discovered or if assessment indicates the medicine is no longer suitable for the patient
- make a clear, accurate and immediate record of all medicines administered, intentionally withheld or refused by the patient
- where supervising a student in the administration of medicines, clearly countersign the signature of the student.

In addition the following may help:

- where possible organise workload and deployment of staff to reduce interruptions during medicine rounds
- prepare medicine in a quiet area
- work with pharmacy to undertake audits to identify where errors occur and ask for additional training in these areas
- take time to keep up to date about the medicines used in your areas and to read your organisations medicines management policy and ask for clarification
- use clinical supervision sessions to discuss your concerns
- if in doubt ask.

Calculations

You should be able to accurately calculate the correct volume or quantity of medicines, for example:

- the rate of flow for IV infusions, ie mls /hour
- the amount based on body weight
- elixirs
- the number of tablets for the dose prescribed.

Sometimes the calculations can be quite complex and if in doubt you should ask a second practitioner to check the calculation (Table 9.1).

Many hospitals offer training session in calculations, especially for newly registered nurses. If you are concerned about calculating medicines you should ask your line manager or pharmacy if they offer any of these sessions.

Covert administration of medicines

This refers to disguising medicines in food and drink. Disguising medication in the absence of informed consent may be regarded as deception. It is only likely to be necessary for patients who actively refuse medication and who are judged not to have the capacity to consent or refuse to consent. The United Kingdom Central Council issued guidance on this in 2001. The key principles for the registered nurse and midwife are:

- ensure what you are doing is in the best interest of the patient
- discuss the proposal with the rest of the multidisciplinary team
- undertake a risk assessment
- consult local policies and guidelines and the United Kingdom Central Council (now NMC) position statement
- seek advice from senior colleagues and the organisation's legal advisors
- document actions and rationale.

Self medication

Self medication of patients in hospital is being seen increasingly as good practice. Studies suggest that it helps improve compliance prior to discharge (Hatch and Tapley, 1982, Bird, 1990) and patients who are able to administer their own medicines were more satisfied with their overall care and with the discharge process. (Deeks et al, 2000). However, where self administration is introduced, arrangements must be in place for the safe secure storage of the medication with access limited to the nurse and the specific patient. In addition, the patient should be periodically assessed to ensure they are still capable of self medicating. If self administration is being used in your organisation there should be a policy to guide you in this practice.

Patient education

Patients must be given information and be educated about their medicines: how and when to take them and what possible side effects to look for. Patients will vary in the amount they want to know, but as a minimum they should be able to make an informed choice about whether to take the medicine, including the consequences of not taking it, and be able to take it safely when they get home. This may involve some supervised practice of self administration while in hospital and possibly the use of compliance aids to help them. Written information may be an important adjunct to verbal explanations and pharmacy colleagues can often help. Relatives may need to be involved in this process.

Table 9.1: Formula used in IM and IV drug calculations

To calculate the volume of solution required to give a prescribed dose of drug by injection the following formula should be used

$$\text{Volume required} = \frac{\text{What you want}}{\text{What you've got}} \times \text{Volume it's in}$$

Example
A patient is prescribed pethidine 75mg by IM injection. This drug is dispensed in ampoules of 100mg in 2 mls

$$\frac{75 \text{ mg}}{100 \text{ mg}} \times 2 = 1.5 \text{ mls}$$

Formula used to calculate IV drip rates

To calculate the rate of infusion the following should be known:

- The number of drops per ml the giving set delivers (standard giving sets deliver 15 ml of blood or blood products per ml of solution and 20 drops of aqueous intravenous fluid per ml of solution). You should check the giving set being used.
- The volume to be administered.
- The time period over which it should be administered.

For manually controlled administration:

$$\text{Infusion rate} = \frac{\text{volume of infusion in mls. x (drop per ml of giving set)}}{\text{Time in minutes}}$$

Example
The prescription requires 1 litre of normal saline to be given in eight hours

$$\text{Infusion rate} = \frac{1000\text{mls (1L) x 20 drop}}{8 \text{ hours x } 60} = \frac{20{,}000}{480} = 41.66 \text{ or 42 drops per minute (rounded up to nearest drop)}$$

Remember what you can do

- As a registered nurse you have responsibility for the safe storage and custody of medicines.
- You should have day to day working knowledge of your medicines management policy or equivalent.
- You should know what action to take of there is a medication error.
- You should seek advice from you pharmacy department if you have any queries.

References

Bird C (1990) A prescription for self-help. *Nurs Times* **86**(43): 52–5

Controls Assurance (2002) Medicines Management (Safe and Secure Handling): 1–33

Crown Report (1998) Review of Prescribing, Supply and Administration of Medicines: a Report on the Supply and Administration of Medicines Under Group Protocols. Department of Health, London

Crown Report (1999) Review of Prescribing, Supply and Administration of Medicines Final Report. Department of Health, London

Deeks P (2000) Are patients who self- administer their medicines in hospital more satisfied with their care. *J AdvNurs* **31**(2): 395–400

Hatch AM, Tapley A (1982) A self administration system for elderly patients at Highbury Hospital. *Nurs Times* **78**: 1773–4

O'Shea E (1999) Factors contributing to medication errors: a literature review. *J Clin Nurs* **8**(5): 496–504

The Medicines Act (1968)

The Misuse of Drugs Act (1971)

NHSLA and Willis (2003) Safe Medicines Practice. *NHS Litigation Authority Review* **27**: 6–9

Nursing and Midwifery (Council 2004) Guidelines for the Administration of Medicines. NMC, London

UKCC (2001) UKCC Position Statement on the Covert Administration of Medicines – Disguising Medicines in Food and Drink. UKCC, London

Additional reading

Audit Commission (2001) A Spoonful of Sugar, Medicines Management in NHS Hospitals

Dimond B (2003) Principles for the correct administration of medicines: 2. *Br J Nurs* **12**(12): 760–2

Dimond B (2003) Patient group directions to enable hospital nurses to supply medicines. *Br J Nurs 12*(14): 880–3

DoH (2004) Building a Safer NHS for Patients: Improving Medication Safety. DoH, London

HSC (200/026) Patient Group Directives(England) NHS Executive

HSC (1998/051) Report on the Supply and Administration of Medicines under Group directives. NHS Executive

Hutton M (1998) Numeracy skills for intravenous calculations. *Nurs Standard* **12**(43): 49–56

Hyde L (2002) Legal and professional aspects of intravenous therapy. *Nurs Standard* **16**(26): 39–42

NMC (2002) Guidelines for the Administration of Medication. NMC, London

Trim J (2004) Clinical skills: a practical guide to working out drug calculations. *Br J Nurs* **13**(10): 602–6

Helpful websites

www.nmc-uk.org   Nursing and Midwifery Council
www.mhra.gov.uk   Medicines and Health care Products
                              Regulatory Agency

www.dh.gov.uk/policyAndGuidance/
    MedicinesPharmacyAndIndustry
    Service/Prescriptions/Nursing
    Prescribing/fs/en   Nurse Prescribing
www.dh.gov.uk/PolicyAndGuidance/
    MedicinesPharmacyAndIndustry
    Services/Prescriptions/Supplementary
    Prescribing/fs/en   Supplementary Prescribing

Chapter 10

Spiritual aspects in hospital nursing

George Castledine

The root meaning of the word 'spiritual' comes from the phenomenon of moving air, breath and wind. It is the animating life force of human beings and may be defined and understood in diverse ways according to different religions and cultural and philosophical traditions. It is not organised religion. It is an integral part of our lives, wherever we go and what ever we do. This chapter aims to help you understand spirituality and how you might help patients with their spirituality. It also suggests pointers to assessing patients' and your own spirituality and how you and your colleagues can develop more spiritual awareness in your workplace. Finally the chapter looks at loss, grief and bereavement in hospital, care of the dying and breaking bad news.

The theoretical and empirical literature identifies four spiritual needs:

- the search for meaning
- a sense of forgiveness
- the need for love
- a need for hope.

(Ronaldson 1997)

Any crisis or moving encounter can trigger our spiritual awareness. However, we may only pause for a few moments' thought or reflection and then push the experience to the back of our minds. In recent years both the medical and nursing professions have become lost and too focused on materialism, medical technology, functionalism and medical treatment and cure. We assess and treat people as if they were just bodies without souls.

In January 1939, Professor RS Aitken gave an inaugural lecture on the occasion of his appointment to the chair of medicine at Aberdeen University. His key message was that there was a great necessity for doctors, and their patients to become friends. Although intended for doctors this timeless message has great relevance for nurses.

Aitken, like many other great doctors and nurses, makes the point that there is more to patient care than scientific and empirical knowledge of disease. In any major illness, doctors and nurses cannot fully help their patients unless they know something of the patient's temperament, past experiences, hopes, fears and attitudes. Aitken said that the body and mind were interwoven and that a patient's whole life history helps to determine both the effect that the illness has on them. Modern doctors and nurses are in danger of delivering patient care without considering their own or their patients' spirituality. It is essential that nurses develop further the spiritual traditions of past nursing leaders.

Nurses have always subscribed to the view that nursing has a spiritual dimension but have often failed to express it clearly enough in theory and practice. They believe that individuals are more than just the physical aspects of their body and that nursing care is more than the undertaking of a set of functional prescribed tasks and skills related to medical treatment protocols and cure-related activities. Nursing has always resisted stereotypes that define and represent nursing and 'doing'; yet at the beginning of the 21st century, nursing still has the same struggles as those faced by Nightingale and others at the end of the 19th century, eg lack of recognition that nursing is a unique practice rather than a set of tasks.

Being the patient's 'friend' and helping them with their spirituality is not a new concept. However, it is an aspect of nursing and medicine that needs reinforcing and not forgetting.

Assessing the patient's spirituality

Here are some key points to bear in mind:

- be sensitive and listen
- don't be judgemental
- be aware of yourself and be reflective
- consider whether the patient's spirituality is linked to a religious framework such as God or a deity whose teaching is followed
- consider whether the patient's spirituality non religious but based on other factors
- remember that spiritual need is unique and is very much determined by the individual
- consider whether the patient is angry, distressed, fearful or preoccupied with suffering and death

The nursing assessment of the patient's spiritual needs is very rarely carried out. There are probably many reasons for this, including the assessing nurse's embarrassment at having to ask the question. Sometimes what the patient says seems so private and personal that the assessing nurse feels it is too sensitive to write down.

Spiritual assessment is difficult, especially in a very busy acute hospital. Stoll (1979) gives us some guidelines. Ask the patient:

- is religion or God significant to you?
- if yes in what ways?
- is prayer helpful?
- would you like to see a hospital chaplain during your stay with us?
- who is the most important person or animal to you?
- to whom do you turn in times of need?
- has your illness /injury made you more aware of yourself and what the consequences might be?

Assessing one's own spirituality.

- Try and reflect about the meaning of life and the effect dying patients have on you.
- Sit quietly listening to music and meditate.
- Reflect how you feel when on a walk in the countryside.
- How are you influenced by certain buildings and churches?
- Record in your diary what makes a good or bad day.

Encouraging more spiritual awareness in the workplace

Hospitals are organisations which often seem to be vibrant and caring places. Many people are born in them, work in them and die in them. They have developed through the centuries into spectacular buildings, full of modern technology and intensive treatment centres. Today, however, hospitals are rapidly evolving from being highly valued centres of acute and rehabilitative clinical care to very expensive cost centres concerned only with the acute aspects of medical treatment. In the past, hospitals had time to nurse patients and allow them to recover properly before they were transferred, if necessary to appropriate places for convalescence.

The intensity with which patients are nursed and treated in hospitals is more pressurised than ever before. Tightly managed and captive environments cause every patient intervention and action to be closely scrutinised as to cost and evidence-based medical care. The race is on from the moment of admission to treat patients and get them home as soon as possible.

The hospital is now becoming more and more like any other big business institution or organisation. It is in danger of losing its soul. Briskin (1998) points out that the modern day workplace and organisation has resulted in the loss of individuals being allowed or able to cultivate their own sense of purpose and direction at work. Efficiency, targets and outcomes have given senior managers total control and dominance over work processes and made workers dependent on management to dictate the terms of their employment. Briskin (1998) calls for the need to humanise the workplace and put some form of soul back into organisations.

Studies in North America have now found that executives see spirituality as very important and a key issue in determining an organisation's performance.

Many people believe strongly that organisations must harness the immense spiritual energy within each person in order to produce world-class products and services.

(McGeachy, 2001)

There are believed to be many characteristics which emerge as personal or individual expressions of spirituality at work. These are:

- searching for 'truth' and meaning while at work
- taking personal responsibility for one's life
- finding meaning and purpose to life outside work
- personal satisfaction
- internal motivatation
- using all aspects of self to full potential
- self knowledge and authenticity
- ability to face fear and death.

The importance of recognising spirituality in people is that the workplace becomes more sensitive and looks after its workers. A strong sense of 'we' is developed instead of 'I', because each person knows that they are appreciated and valued. It is therefore important that hospitals develop the concept of spirituality in the workplace. Perhaps, if this happened more, there would be a greater inter-professional health team understanding and working together for the patient.

Suggestions to stimulate spiritual intelligence in the hospital:

- Run workshops on intuition, meditation, stress relief, active and deep listening, creativity and tai chi.

- Listen to what spirituality means for all members of the health team.
- Ask people to identify the critical issues for them at work and the ways they cope with them.
- Encourage people to express their spirituality and talk about ways they can develop themselves at work.
- Provide development training for staff and encourage life-long learning and personal development at work.
- Make work fun, and have special days to celebrate team work.

Loss, grief and bereavement in hospital

Regardless of age, sex, creed and culture, the experience of grief in response to loss is known to all human beings. It is a fact of life.

(Sanders, 1989)

Grief is a descriptive word which tries to indicate the state the person is in and the range of psychological, physical and emotional reactions to loss. Extremes of grief appear when one loses a close and meaningful relationship. Death, divorce, separation, abortion, the loss of a limb, bodily function or lifestyle will precipitate this most painful human emotion.

Bereavement is a blanket term used to describe the whole event and vast array of emotions, experiences, changes and conditions that take place as a result of loss and grief reactions. The length of time an individual spends in bereavement depends on many things, such as, the intensity of the relationship, and whether death was anticipated or not.

Whatever the cause of the loss, there is little value in carers and nurses making comparisons about the feelings they have. There is no consolation in hearing that there is always someone worse off than you.

The feelings people experience when they are bereaved are healthy, normal and part of the healing process. Failure to express them may often lead to more intensive reactions, such as severe depression and physical illness.

For many carers, especially nurses, it is normal and empathic to feel helpless and unable to find something to say or do that will make the bereaved feel instantly better. 'It's just a matter of time', or 'you'll get over it', are platitudes that are not helpful. What the bereaved person needs from the carer or nurse is the courage to stay and listen to how much it hurts.

Of all the qualities a nurse should possess, perhaps the most important is compassion, particularly when nursing the critically ill and dying. It is not easy to define compassion. Sogyal Rinpoche (1992) a Tibetan monk sums up the term:

> *It is not simply a sense of sympathy or caring for the person*
> *suffering, not simply warmth of heart towards the person before you,*
> *or a sharp clarity of recognition of their needs and pain, it is also a*
> *sustained and practical determination to do whatever is possible and*
> *necessary to help alleviate their suffering.*

Rinpoche also stresses that 'compassion is not true compassion unless it is active'. Therefore, as a nurse, you must seek ways to develop and activate your feelings of compassion.

Throughout the centuries, prayer has been used to focus more clearly and directly on those for whom people are feeling compassion. Florence Nightingale placed great emphasis on prayer. The saying of prayers at the beginning of the day used to be an important ritual and routine of ward nursing.

Over the years, however, this spiritual dimension of nursing care has disappeared. Prayer is now only associated with ministers of religion and religious institutions such as churches, synagogues, mosques and temples.

There is more to prayer than just religious tradition. First, it enables us to reflect on our own mortality. Second, it helps us to relate to our wishes and desires. We only ever seem to turn to prayer when we are troubled, under threat, in need, have achieved something special or if a miraculous thing has happened. The Jewish novelist Isaac Singer once said: 'Whenever I'm in trouble, I pray. Since I'm always in trouble I pray always.' When asked: 'Why are you in trouble?' He replied: 'Who is not in trouble?' (cited in Pritchard, 1998).

Who indeed? Perhaps we all tend to turn to prayer of some kind. Usually it is not religious in nature but an internalised reflection that is the essence of our spiritual selves. When we are charged with caring for people, prayer can help us reflect on our responsibilities, relationships and purpose. Rinpoche (1992) states that prayer can: 'direct whatever compassion you have to all beings, by dedicating all your positive actions and spiritual practice to their welfare and especially their enlightenment.'

It is difficult to understand what is meant by enlightenment, but much emphasis is placed on it in Tibetan tradition and religious practices. Enlightenment comes through experiencing, interacting and reflecting on life. It is the 'calm' untroubled state which many patients seem to achieve when faced with momentous and life threatening situations.

Sometimes it is felt that just because prayer does not produce measured results it is a pointless exercise. Pritchard (1998) suggests that if the question associated with prayer is 'Does it produce the goods?' then we have abandoned the sphere of faith and are ignoring the intuitive and basic elements of prayer.

Prayer should never be imposed on patients or used as a substitute for the nurse's time and presence. A careful and sensitive spiritual assessment of the patient's state is essential. Prayer may facilitate the patients' understanding of themselves, their situation, their spiritual identity, or their relationship with their god or spiritual maker. It is not there to convey a false sense of hope and expectation or penitence.

Prayer can be used to improve our understanding of what is happening around us. Its use as a nursing intervention and a reflection strategy is not new in nursing. However, perhaps the time has come to consider how it can find a place in today's modern healthcare world and to what extent a nurse's spiritual awareness is central to their nursing care.

Care of the dying patient

Patients who are dying require intensive physical, emotional and social support. Their reactions are usually based on their beliefs and previous encounters with death. It is important not to isolate them or leave their families and friends to cope alone.

The physical needs of the patient

This should include regular two-hourly positioning with attention to skin care, toileting and general hygiene and bed linen should be applied loosely to reduce discomfort caused by pressure on arms and legs.

There are two phases of dying which occur before the actual time of death: the pre-active phase and the active phase of dying. Sometimes it is very difficult to detect when one phase leads into another or when there is a subtle difference in the change. The pre-active phase usually lasts about two to three weeks and the active phase three to four days.

Signs and symptoms of the pre-active phase are:

1. withdrawal from social activities and events in the immediate environment
2. tiredness and lack of energy
3. loss of appetite
4. breathing changes with periods of apnoea or absence
5. possible fluid retention and oedema
6. loss of weight
7. susceptibility to chest infections
8. skin breakdown if not carefully attended to
9. dryness of mouth and a need for regular oral hygiene

10. changes in bowels or bladder function.

Signs and symptoms of the active phase are:

1. changes in the depth and rate of respiration
2. very low blood pressure
3. weak and thready pulse rate
4. change in skin temperature
5. decreased level of consciousness
6. changes in sensation and neuromuscular control
7. changes in appearance – pallor
8. cyanosis
9. sweating – sometimes heavy (diaphoresis)
10. skin changes eg. mottling.

Emotional and psychological changes are often dependent upon the character and individual differences of each patient. It is sometimes very difficult to predict how someone will cope with dying. In the very early stages of death some patients feel they want to accomplish something and put their personal business affairs in order.

Factors that influence coping with death

- the age of the person
- past and present personal experiences associated with loss and dying
- religious and spiritual background
- culture, ethnicity and society
- self awareness, character and degree of acceptance by the individual of mortality
- family and close friends.

It is believed that there are several stages which the dying person passes through. The most acceptable description of these are the five psychological stages described by Elizabeth Kübler-Ross (1975). Although research has shown that not all patients experience these states or go through them in the same way, they act as a useful guide in nursing assessment.

Stage	Characteristics	Nursing tips
1 Denial	(Following a diagnosis of terminal illness) 'No'. Shock, numbness, refusal to accept diagnosis, sweating, tachycardia, gastric disorders, fainting	Be honest and support the patient Keep in close contact Encourage the patient to talk Don't push or force acceptance of the diagnosis
2 Anger	'Why me?' Resentment, feelings of loss of control over life, aggression, shouting and blaming others	Maintain contact Keep calm Don't antagonise Be supportive and present if need be
3 Bargaining	'Can I trade?' Acknowledgement, feelings of trading and swapping things for more time	Support and listen Don't insist on the patient keeping the results of their bargaining
4 Reactive depression	'I am dying, leave me alone.' Feelings of desperation, sleep upset and other classic signs of a depressive state. Grieving about a situation, withdrawal, anorexia, stress fatigue, self neglect and tearfulness	Encourage patient to talk Listen, provide comfort and support Resist temptation to be over optimistic but don't deny hope
5 Acceptance	'Okay! Let me sort my life out and my affairs.' Accepts the inevitable, without being overly emotional or stressed. Wants friendship and reality – someone who cares and is realistic	Be there if the patient wants you Help and support in sorting out business and family matters Encourage communication and listen to what the patient wants

In summary the needs of the dying person are:

Physical Essential care and nursing of daily living activites and needs Good symptom control 'Palliation' Comfort Relaxing and stress free environment	Emotional/Psychological Hope Respect Self-control Inter-dependence with nurses and carers Honesty and open communication A listener Empathy Holism Individual personal care
Social Time to put life and business in order Home adaptations Possible special aids to daily living Presence of close friends and family Community recognition for privacy and dignity	Spiritual Expression of own individual beliefs and practices Forgiveness, reconciliation Spiritual process at death Peace and understanding of self-situation

When someone dies – practical matters

There are several key things which must be considered by the relations or those representing the dead person.

1. Any special requests or religious/ cultural practices for laying out and dealing with the body. The nurse's role is often to carry out "last offices" or laying out the body. The body should usually be left for an hour before last offices is carried out. This will involve:
   - bathing the body
   - laying it flat and wrapping it in a shroud
   - reviewing the hospital policy regarding any particular procedures
   - replacing dentures
   - removing any tubes, catheters and infusions
   - if leakage is present from wounds or orifices, packing or padding according to policy
   - expressing the bladder into a receiver if necessary
   - removing all jewellery from the body, unless advised otherwise, or taping into position
   - fitting the shroud and fastening carefully
   - ensure that name bands and labels are completed accurately and applied correctly
   - wrapping the body in a sheet and securing with tape
   - two nurses carefully packing the patient's belongings and securing any valuables according to the trust policy
   - taking the body to the hospital mortuary.
2. Funeral directors should be contacted.
3. The death should be registered at the local register office and the following items will be necessary:
   - the medical certificate of the cause of death
   - the deceased person's medical card
   - the deceased person's birth certificate or passport.
4. In some circumstances (eg sudden death) the coroner may need to be informed.
5. The deceased's solicitor needs to be contacted.
6. Other services or agencies and organisations need to be informed of the death.

Most hospitals now have special bereavement officers who deal with bereaved relatives and the removal of the body from the hospital mortuary. Usually any relatives or close friends have the right to view the body and this takes place in the appropriate viewing room or chapel of rest.

Dealing with the bereaved

There is no 'right' way to grieve. Therefore the nurse needs to be aware of the general principles and allow for individual variations. Some people are able to carry on almost normally, while others may feel for a time that they and the world are falling apart. Bereavement takes time and may follow through various stages, some identifiable, others merging into one another.

Emotional reactions

- numbness, shock
- denial
- pining and despair
- depression
- guilt
- anger
- anxiety

Physical reactions

- not eating
- not sleeping
- bodily distress – gastro-intestinal, dyspepsia, heartburn, constipation
- migraine
- acute chest pain

Viewing the body

Many people do not 'want' or 'like' to see the dead body of someone they love. However, there is good evidence to suggest that, if they are supported and receive positive comments, the experience will be less traumatic and may even help them in accepting the person's death.

It is important to prepare relatives before they view the body:

- Describe the scene and what to expect in the room.
- Explain how the body will look.
- Encourage the bereaved to talk about the experience and to the dead person's body.

- Don't hurry the bereaved; take time and be present with them.

Supporting the bereaved

Remember the following general points to help the bereaved come to terms with their loss:

- Listen actively.
- Encourage expression of feelings; give permission to grieve.
- Let them cry.
- Encourage them to talk about the dead person.
- Support their coping mechanisms and let them express themselves as individuals.
- Express your sorrow and share your feeling with them.
- Encourage them to be patient – 'it takes time'.
- Reassure them and involve them in what is happening in the wider world. Don't isolate them by thinking it is a better if they are left alone.
- Put them in contact with local support agencies if necessary such as Cruse Bereavement Care or local counselling.
- Encourage the person to get back into a regular routine, to adopt a good diet and wait for a while before throwing away personal belongings of the dead person.

Breaking bad news

'Bad news' can be defined as any information that drastically alters a patient's view of their future for the worse.

The nurse should think carefully before giving bad news to people. It is a very important skill and requires the practitioner to be fully aware of how they may possibly react themselves in similar circumstances.

It is important when giving bad news to interlace facts with questions such as: 'How do you feel about what I've just said?' In addition it is important to give the receiver time to reflect on what you have said.

Preparation is very important – know all the facts and prepare for the meeting.

- The environment should ensure privacy and be very comfortable.
- Have tissues ready and warm or cold drinks.

- Ask questions, first about what the individual knows.
- Clarify information.
- Give warning shots such as, 'I'm very sorry but this looks serious'.
- Allow the patient to deny things; be aware how much information they can cope with.
- Keep it simple; details will not be remembered.
- Listen and show your willingness to deal with their reactions.
- Encourage them to ventilate and express their feelings. Allow them to cry if necessary.
- At the end of the session, summarise and review key points and plans for the future.
- Offer to be available for further clarification and support.
- Evaluate how you think you coped with it all and review your performance during clinical supervision.

Remember what you can do

- Reflect on how well you help patients with their spirituality.
- Discuss with colleagues how you can incorporate an assessment of spirituality into your current assessment process.
- Ask for support and help from senior colleagues, chaplains and others.
- Try using the suggestions to assess your own spirituality.
- Consider how you express, or would like to express, spirituality at work and how this affects the work you do.
- Consider how others express spirituality and how this impacts on you and your colleagues.
- With colleagues, suggest ways to stimulate spirituality in the hospital.
- Reflect on the care you have given to patients dying in hospital and consider how you might have approached this differently now you have read this chapter.

References

Aitken RS (1939) Making a competent physician. *Aberdeen Press and Journal*, Friday 13 January: 6

Briskin A (1998) The Stirring of the Soul in the Workplace. Berrett- Koehler Pubs, San Fransisco

Kubler Ross E (1975) Death – the Final Stages of Growth. Prentice Hall, Englewood Cliffs

McGeachy C (2001) Spiritual Intelligence in the Workplace. Veritus Pubs, Dublin

Pritchard J (1998) The Intercessions Handbook. 2nd edition. SPCK, London

Ronaldson S (1997) Spirituality: the Heart of Nursing. Ausmed Pub, Melbourne

Rinpoche S (1992) The Tibetan Book of Living and Dying. Random House, London: 187–201

Sanders CM (1989) Grief, the Mourning after Dealing with Adult Bereavement. John Wiley and Sons, New York

Stoll R (1979) Guidelines for spiritual assessment. *Am J Nurs* 79: 1574–7

Additional reading

Carson VB (1989) Spiritual Dimensions of Nursing Practice. WB Saunders Co, Philadelphia

Castledine G (1998) The value of prayer in modern-day nursing. *Br J Nurs* 7(20): 1290

Castledine G (2000) Spirituality and being a friend of the patient. *Br J Nurs* 9(1): 62

Cruse Bereavement Care – An international journal published three times a year Edited by Dr Colin Murray Parkes and Dr Dora Black. Published by Cruse Bereavement Care

Cruse Bereavement Care – After the Death of Someone Very Cose. Cruse Bereavement Care, Richmond Surrey

Cooke H (2000) When Someone Dies. Butterworth. Heinemann, Oxford

Copp G (1998) A review of current theories of death and dying. *J Adv Nurs* 28(2): 382–90

Dickenson D, Johnson M, Samson Katz J (2000) Death Dying and Bereavement. 2nd edition. Open University and Sage Publications, London

Haas F (2003) Bereavement care seeing the body. *Nurs Standard* 17(28): 33–7

Kelly P (1979) Companion to grief. Piatkus, London

Longaker C (1997) Facing Death and Finding Hope. Century, London

McNamara B (2001) Fragile Lives – Death Dying and Care. Open University Press, Buckingham

Murrey-Parkes C (1986) Bereavement Studies of Grief in Adult Life. Penguin, Harmondsworth

NHS Scotland (2002) Guidelines on Chaplaincy and Spiritual Care in the NHS and Scotland. NHS HDL 2002, 76 Scottish Executive, Edinburgh

Quested B (2003) Nursing care of dead bodies: a discursive analysis of last offices. *J Adv Nurs* 41(6) 553–60

Scrutton S (1995) Bereavement and Grief, Supporting Older People through Loss. Cruse and Age Concern, London

Tanyi R (2002) Towards clarification of the meaning of spirituality. *J Adv Nurs* **39**(5): 500–9

Helpful websites

www.cruseberavementcare.org.uk   Cruse Bereavement Care

Section 2
The importance of the patient's environment

The importance of the patient's environment

Our surroundings affect us for better or worse and when people are unwell the environment really does matter. It has to provide comfort and a background and facilities that will help patients get better. Nowadays patients expect high quality care in hospitals that are clean, tidy, well organised and welcoming. It gives them more confidence in the staff and services provided.

The state of many hospitals buildings has been poor for many years with a lack of maintenance, refurbishment and repairs. However in more recent years there has been an increase in the number of new hospitals built as a result of Private Finance Initiatives and there have been resources targeted specifically at the hospital environment through the Clean Hospitals Environment Programme (NHS Estates 2001) in order to improve the environment. This is essential if patients are to be cared for in an aesthetically pleasing, light and airy environment which provides a feeling of space. Pictures and colours can provide interest and at the same time convey a feeling of peacefulness.

Hospitals also need to be 'user friendly' places. Patients need to be able to find the ward or department they are looking for and therefore signposting should be clear and accurate. Many patients have to travel some distance or they may be disabled. Parking in hospitals all over the country is problematic and this adds to patients and relatives worry and anxiety when coming to hospital. They need to be confident that they can park near to the hospital or at least be able to be dropped off near to the department they are attending.

Florence Nightingale is famous for stating, 'the hospital shall do the patient no harm'. However ensuring the safety of everyone that comes into contact with health services is one of the most important challenges. It is known there are at least a million incidents, accidents and errors occurring in the NHS each year. Hospitals must be able to protect patients, visitors and staff and minimise the risk of things going wrong by learning from mistakes.

Although many of the problems of the patients' environment are beyond the scope of one individual to remedy, there are many things that you can do to make the patients' environment safe, secure and welcoming and this section highlights these.

Chapter 11 Health and Safety summarises key aspects of health and safety legislation relevant to you in your work and identifies common hazards you will encounter in your work and the systems that need to be put in place to minimise risks. *Chapter 12 Medical Devices* explains the regulations that have been introduced to minimise the risk of using medical devices and highlights the responsibility of nursing staff. *Chapter 13 Infection control* examines the nature of hospital acquired infections and the role of the nurse in preventing and controlling these. Finally *Chapter 14 Assessing and managing the patient's environment* focuses on how the clinical environment should be assessed and managed to make sure it meets legislation and is safe and secure for patients and visitors and that it is an appropriate working environment for staff.

References

NHS Estates (2001) *National Standards of cleanliness for NHS.* NHS Estates Executive Organisation of the DOH: London

Chapter 11

Health and safety

Ann Close

This chapter summarises the key aspects of health and safety legislation relevant to nurses in hospital and identifies common hazards and the systems that need to be put in place to control and minimise the risks.

Health and Safety legislation

Health in the workplace is regulated by the Department of Employment and not the Department of Health. The Health and Safety Commission and its operational arm the Health and Safety Executive (HSE) are the main agents for enforcing health and safety at work and they have a statutory remit to inspect all work premises and enforce health and safety legislation. They have the power to issue improvement notices to employers and serious offences may lead to prosecution.

The Health and Safety at Work Act was introduced in 1974 and set out the duties of employers and employees in ensuring health and safety at work. All public and private health sector employers are covered by the legislation.

For employers there is a requirement to:

- Ensure, so far as is reasonably possible, the health, safety and welfare at work of all employees. This is extended to include people who, although are not employees, use the premises, such as patients, their visitors, the public and any contracted workers.

Employees have a duty to:

- Take reasonable care of their own health and safety and that of others who may be affected by their acts or omissions at work. This requires employees to assist employers with health and safety matters by doing such things as notifying them of serious and imminent dangers and using equipment and safe systems of work provided by the employer.

European directives

In 1992 the European directives were implemented. The purpose of these directives was to provide codes of practice and practical guidance for ensuring health and safety at work. They consisted of a 'six pack':

- The approved code of practice for the **management of health and safety at work**. These regulations set out broad general duties which apply to all kinds of work. They include the need to assess risks so that the necessary preventive and protective measures can be taken and a requirement to provide health surveillance, information and training.
- The approved code of practice for **workplace health, safety and welfare**. These regulations set the general requirements for:
  - the working environment including such things as temperature, lighting, ventilation and workstations
  - safety - including safety of the buildings and surroundings such as safe opening of doors and windows, safety of passengers and vehicles, prevention of falls from heights or injury from falling objects
  - facilities – including the provision of toilets, washing, eating and changing facilities, rest areas and facilities for pregnant and nursing mothers
  - housekeeping – including maintenance of the workplace, equipment, cleanliness and the removal of waste materials.
- Guidance on regulations for **work equipment**. These regulations place general duties on employers and list minimum requirements for work equipment which is defined as anything from a hand tool to machines of all kinds. This will therefore include medical devices, wheel chairs, commodes, computers, beds and many more.
- Guidance on regulations for **personal protective equipment at work**. These are the regulations regarding all equipment including clothing that is intended to be worn or held by people which protects them against one or more risks to their health and safety. It includes clothes such as aprons, gloves and safety footwear and equipment such as eye protectors, and lead jackets.
- Guidance on regulations for **manual handling**. These regulations require avoidance of manual handling operations as far as possible by using an alternative approach or using mechanical or electrical equipment. It also requires that assessments of manual handling operations are undertaken.
- Guidance on regulations for **display screen equipment work**. This includes the need for analysis of workstations and risk assessments of the environment to ensure that lighting is appropriate without reflections and glare.

The control of substances hazardous to health COSHH (HSE, 1994)

These regulations cover any form of substance including micro-organisms and allergens that are able to damage health through being absorbed, injected, inhaled or ingested. They place a duty on the employer and its employees to protect all persons in the workplace against immediate or delayed risks of substances hazardous to health. They require employers to report any infections attributable to work including exposure to blood, body fluids or infected materials.

Fire safety

Hospitals are particularly vulnerable to fire and the Secretary of State expects each NHS organisation to have a clearly defined fire precautions policy and a satisfactory level of physical fire precautions designed to prevent the occurrence, ensure the detection and stop the spread of fire. The hospital should be able to:

- raise the alarm
- fight a fire
- move or evacuate patients in an emergency
- train staff in all these matters.

Actions to take in the event of a fire are included in *Chapter 6.*

Common hazards in the workplace

A hazard is something that has the potential to cause harm. Although every ward, department and hospital will have its unique health and safety risks, there are a number of common hazards that will be present in every area. These include:

Lifting and handling

The health risks of lifting and handling patients and other loads are well known. Back pain among nursing staff costs the NHS considerable sums of money through sick leave, temporary replacement staff, treatment costs and compensation claims and there are varying degrees of suffering for the individual concerned. Dangerous methods of lifting and lack of proper equipment are the main causes of back injury. Problems are usually due to cumulative long term effects rather than a single event and the most hazardous manoeuvres are the manual transfer of patients between bed and chair, manual repositioning of patients in bed and lifting patients in and out of the bath. Other pre-disposing factors to back pain are job satisfaction, relationships with colleagues, stress levels and the way in which work is organised (Moffet et al, 1993).

Although safer policies are in place in most NHS organisations, together with training programmes, two thirds of trusts believe that nurses are not complying due to peer pressure from other nurses, staff shortages, lack of time, lack of equipment and lack of supervision (Parish, 2002).

Biological hazards.

These may result from:

- Needlestix injuries: In health care blood borne viruses such as hepatitis B and C and HIV are most commonly transmitted as a result of percutaneous exposure following sharps injuries.
- Clinical waste: Giving rise to bacteria in the healthcare environment from secretions, excretions and bed linen.

Chemical hazards

These may be caused by disinfectants, solvents and other cleaning agents. The risks of gluteraldehyde exposure are well known. It is commonly used in endoscopy units, theatres, dental and ENT departments and outpatients to sterilise fibre optic endoscopes, laryngeal mirrors or for equipment that requires rapid turn round times. The common hazards of exposure are dermatitis, asthma and eye irritation. Latex allergies are also hazards and can cause hypersensitivity and result in dermatitis.

Violence and aggression

Although this is not a new problem, the incidence and severity appears to be increasing. Violence and aggression can be experienced by a wide range of staff groups in hospitals and the community but there is a higher risk to ambulance staff, nurses, accident and emergency staff and those caring for people with behavioural problems. Physical injuries as a result of violence are obvious but continuous exposure to verbal abuse may adversely affect health as a result of stress.

Occupational stress

Guidance from the Health and Safety Executive (HSE, 2001) informs employers of their legal duty to ensure their employees are not made ill by their work as a result of increasing pressure and change. Bullying and harassment also add to stress levels. The HSE estimates that workers take 13.4 million days off a year in the UK because of stress and there is evidence that employees in health professions are suffering more stress than others (Kelly et al, 1995). This can lead to increased time off, high staff turnover, unsafe behaviour and increased accidents.

Managing Health and Safety

Employers are duty bound to protect the health of their employees. They have a legal obligation to identify, assess and take action to reduce and control risks.

This process is applicable whatever type of hazard and the following steps should be followed.

Risk identification

Risks can arise from any of the activities or tasks undertaken on a day-to-day basis, for example, storage and administration of drugs, naso- gastric feeding, cannulation, venepuncture and disposal of clinical waste or from working relationships with colleagues and patients.

Risk assessment

This involves assessing:

- what could go wrong?

- how could it go wrong?
- what are the consequences if it does go wrong – how severe will the harm be?
- what is the likelihood or frequency of it going wrong?

Ratings for severity and likelihood can be made, for example:

Figure 11.1

Likelihood	Consequence				
	Insignificant	Minor	Moderate	Major	Catastrophic
Almost certain	low risk	low risk	moderate risk	high risk	high risk
Likely	low risk	low risk	moderate risk	high risk	high risk
Possible	very low risk	low risk	moderate risk	high risk	high risk
Unlikely	very low risk	very low risk	low risk	moderate risk	high risk
Rare	very low risk	very low risk	low risk	moderate risk	high risk

Both the likelihood and potential consequence ratings are plotted on the following matrix to give an overall rating.

For example:

- If the likelihood of something occurring is almost certain and the consequence or effect is catastrophic such as death then the risk is high.
- If the likelihood of something occurring is possible and the consequence or outcome is minor then the risk is low.

The above scoring system will help to determine the highest and most urgent risks so that priorities can be addressed first.

Reducing and controlling the risk

There may already be controls in place, for example there may be policies, procedures or training. The extent to which these control the risk should be assessed and whether other actions should be taken.

Controls are likely to include:

- **Policies**: which take account of legislation and guide staff on what they should do, how they should act and what their responsibilities are.
- **Safe systems of work**: including safe devices and procedures for staff to follow.

- **Availability of appropriate personal protective clothing**: and sufficient supervision to ensure that staff wear and use these appropriately with sanctions if they do not.
- **Provision of information**: to raise awareness and understanding about the potential effects of the risks, for example ensuring staff understand the long term effects of exposure to gluteraldehyde or the cumulative effects of poor manual handling techniques.
- **Instruction and training**: so that staff are able to understand the policies and have the skills and knowledge to undertake risk assessments and implement the safe systems of work.
- **Systems for monitoring exposure or incidents**: to determine if the controls are working and including such things as, the number of sharps injuries, the levels of gluteraldeyhde in the atmosphere, or the number and type of back injuries.
- **Monitoring the health of employees**: through occupational health checks to determine if there are any emerging problems.

Monitoring and reviewing the assessment

This will determine if the controls put in place have helped to reduce the likelihood of the risk happening and the severity of damage.

Recording the risk assessment

Organisations have different ways of recording risks and developing a risk register. A copy of the risk assessment, controls and outcome of reviews should be kept at both local level and at directorate or organisational level.

Other measures to improve health and safety.

- Staff should be encouraged to discuss hazards in their workplace. They understand the details of what they do and what can go wrong. By involving them they will take more responsibility for health and safety problems.
- There should be a systematic and comprehensive review of the workplace, practices and techniques to identify those which predispose to significant risks.

- The safe systems of work developed should be practical and practicable.
- In some instances pre-employment assessment of an individual or immunisation may be necessary or, in other cases, redeployment of staff may be required.
- Safety representatives: are union members who volunteer to monitor safety and sometimes environmental hazards in the workplace. They deal with issues raised by colleagues and discuss with managers ways of resolving these. They also work with the health and safety committee.

Remember what you can do

- To discharge your responsibilities and duties under health and safety legislation.
- Find out:
  - who the hospital's health and safety officer is and how to contact them
  - if there are any safety representatives working in your area and where you can contact them
  - what the hospital's and the ward/department's policies are on health and safety and where are they kept
  - what risk assessments have been done in your area and where they are kept
  - what the biggest risks are for your areas of work and what you need to do to minimise them
  - what equipment is available and how and when it should be used to reduce risks
  - what training is available and how you can attend
  - how you report an incident, accident, hazard or risk that you have identified
  - if there is any information about the incidents or accidents that have occurred in your area. Are there any trends?
  - what help and support is available from the occupational health service
  - if there is a health and safety circle or similar forum for discussing health and safety issues

References

Health and Safety Executive (1992)
    Management of Health and Safety at Work Regulations
    Workplace Health Safety and Welfare Regulations
    Personal Protective Equipment at Work Regulations
    Provision and Use of Work Equipment Regulations
    Manual Handling Operations Regulations
    Health and Safety (display Screen) Regulations. HMSO, London
Health and Safety Executive (1994) The Control of Substances Hazardous to Health
    Regulations. HMSO, London
Health and Safety Executive (2001) A Manager's guide to Improving and Maintaining
    Employee Health and Wellbeing (HSG 218). HSE, Sudbury
HMSO (1974) Health and Safety at Work Act 1974. HMSO, London
Kelly S et al (1995) Suicide deaths in England and Wales 1982–1992, the contribution
    of occupation and geography. *Population Trends* **80**: 16–25
Moffet JAK, Hughes GI, Griffiths P (1993) A longitudinal study of low back pain in
    student nurses. *J Nurs Stud* **30**(3): 197–212
Parish C (2002) Trusts claim nurses still used banned techniques. *Nurs Standard*
    16(49): 7

Additional reading

Clough J (1998) Assessing and Controlling risk. *Nurs Standard* **12**(31): 49–54
Dimond B (2002) Responsibilities in relation to controlling hazardous substances. *Br
    J Nurs* **11**(14): 941–3
Dimond B (2003) Update and overview of the law relating to health and safety. *Br J
    Nurs* **12**(6): 365–8
Dinsdale P (2003) *Take the danger out of working. Nurs Standard* **17**(34): 12–13
HSE (1999) Guidance and Code of Practice on COSHH. The Stationery Office,
    London

Useful websites

www.hse.gov.uk   Health and Safety Executive
www.dh.gov.uk   Department of Health

Chapter 12

Medical devices

Derek Eaves

During the last twenty-five years, just as our ordinary lives have been transformed by technology with the introduction of personal computers, automatic bank machines, dvds and so on, healthcare has also embraced a variety of equipment to aid diagnosis, treatment and care. The latter have certainly benefited both patients and staff but, not surprisingly, medical devices do not come without dangers. For instance:

> *In 2003 in England and Wales, 87 people died and 558 were seriously injured through incidents with medical devices.*

This may not seem a high number, but it means that, on average at least one patient expecting to be cared for actually dies or is seriously injured every day through misuse of, or malfunctioning, equipment. In addition, every hospital risk manager can give you examples of over-infusion of fluids and drugs, with a range of adverse outcomes, due to user error or as a result of damaged equipment.

This chapter explains what medical devices are, and how regulation has been introduced to minimise their risks and highlights the responsibilities of nursing staff for medical devices used in their work.

What are medical devices?

A medical device is any instrument, apparatus, appliance, material or health care product, excluding drugs, that is used for a patient or client. It is worth reminding yourself of the whole range:

- **For the diagnosis or treatment of disease, or monitoring of patients** eg. dressings, IV administration sets and pumps, implantable defibrillators and pacemakers, patient monitoring equipment, radiology equipment.
- **For critical care** eg. ventilators, defibrillators.

- **In the care of people with disabilities** eg. wheelchairs, pressure relieving equipment.
- **For daily living** eg. commodes, incontinence products, hearing aids etc.
- **In vitro diagnostic devices** eg. devices for blood glucose, pregnancy test kits etc.

Regulation of medical devices

As a result of adverse incidents and recognised risks to patients over the last five years there have been many directives to hospitals regarding medical devices.

Controls assurance standards

Controls assurance standards have been developed to cover many aspects of service provision including medical devices. Hospitals have greatly improved their general systems for managing devices due to this initiative, which has set standards for hospitals to follow mainly on the purchasing, use and maintenance of equipment and training for staff.

The Clinical Negligence Scheme for Trusts (CNST)

The clinical negligence insurance scheme, covering all hospitals in England (and its equivalent in Wales), has directed hospitals to improve their systems for training staff in the use of medical devices.

Medicines and healthcare products

The Medicines and Healthcare Products Regulatory Agency (MHRA) came into existence in 2003 and was derived from two existing bodies, the Medicines Control Agency (MCA) and the Medical Devices Agency (MDA). When hospitals encounter any problems with either drugs or equipment they have to report to this national body, which collates the information and sends out notices and warnings back to all hospitals about any dangerous device or drug.

National Patient Safety Agency

Also, in 2003, the newly formed National Patient Safety Agency (NPSA) declared its interest in reducing risks to patients by improving the use of medical devices. In the first instance, it has decided, in conjunction with the manufacturers to look at the design of devices. For instance, like household appliances, many medical devices have a host of potential settings and programmes when, in fact, some devices only need one or two settings. The reduction in available options could improve safety as, in effect, there is less to go wrong.

Of particular interest to nurses, the NPSA has started an infusion device project, which is presently being piloted at a number of trusts. This includes an infusion device usability evaluation questionnaire, a purchasing checklist to promote good purchasing practice, a document providing advice on how to develop an equipment library and an interactive web-based training package.

Responsibilities of nurses

The key principles nurses should remember are that a medical device should be:

- suitable for its intended purpose
- properly understood by the professional user
- maintained in a safe and reliable condition.

Accountability structures

Each organisation is required to have clear lines of accountability for the use of medical devices. There will be board level responsibility but your ward or department will also have a designated person, usually the ward/department manager, who is accountable for the medical devices in your area. These organisational responsibilities mean that local ward/departmental systems need to be in place for the safe storage, monitoring and proper functioning of the device and staff training. Individual nurses should make sure they are aware of these systems and, if they are either unhappy with their robustness or, more worryingly, discover they do not in fact exist, they should be raising their concerns with their seniors.

It is important to note that if you are using a medical device you are responsible for ensuring you know how to use it and that it is safe for you to use on that particular patient.

Policies

Each organisation is required to have policies for the purchase, acceptance, decontamination, maintenance, replacement and training in the use of medical devices. These are intended to guide you in their safe use.

- Purchasing of equipment should follow the MHRA Medicines and Healthcare Product Regulatory Agency and National Audit Office (NAO) recommendations and this is why it is important that you follow the procurement department's procedures.
- Acceptance checks should be carried out before the equipment is put into use so that its safety can be checked.
- Manufacturers' recommendations should be followed for decontamination which needs to be undertaken after each use and also before the device is returned for servicing or repair. It should be clear whether or not the device is for single use. If it is, then it should not under any circumstance be reused.
- There should be a programme for planned preventative maintenance which should follow manufacturers' instructions.
- There should be an agreed policy for replacement to ensure the equipment is safe and there should be maintenance contracts included in the purchase.
- Users of the equipment need to be trained to use it safely.

Staff training

Nurses have to become knowledgeable about many of the devices mentioned, obviously some more than others. They need to know the basic principles on which the device works and how to use each particular model. The 'bottom line' is that no one should operate any piece of equipment without the correct training. In the past, nurses would arrive on a ward or in a department and any training that did exist tended to be very haphazard. Nurses not properly trained would then pass on incomplete knowledge to others. As well as increasing the risks to patients, this resulted in the majority of equipment being returned to hospital engineering departments as being 'faulty', when, in fact, it worked perfectly well in the hands of knowledgeable staff.

Now hospitals have much more formal arrangements in training staff on equipment. All nurses should familiarise themselves with the training systems in place at their hospital. Normally this will be done as part of a local induction programme. Wards and departments will have access to either written or electronic device instructions, medical device policies, procedures and training programmes and they should be keeping systematic records of all training undertaken. Some hospitals have systems where nurses in each area become local trainers of the rest of the staff, while in some organisations more central training systems will be in place.

As well as ensuring that staff are trained in the use of medical devices, patients and carers (known as 'end users') also have to be trained in the use of the medical devices and any precautions they need to take.

Prior to using any device, it is worth asking yourself the following questions:

- Are you aware of the differences between models of a given device? *– Some devices look exactly the same except for a variation in colour.*
- Do you know how to set the controls effectively? *– Make sure you have set the device to run over one day not one hour for instance.*
- Can you link the device properly to the patient? *– The height of the device relative to the patient may affect infusion rate.*
- Are you able to show the patient how to use the device? *– A knowledgeable patient is a safer patient.*
- Can you recognise malfunctioning of the device? *– The earlier one picks up a problem the less likely it is there will be an adverse outcome.*
- Do you know what to do if a device malfunctions? *– It may not just be a case of stopping the infusion pump - you may have to disconnect it altogether.*
- Do you know who to contact if you are suspicious of malfunction? *– All hospitals will have a nominated person who should be told immediately of any 'near miss' or actual incident.*
- Do you know how to report in writing an incident? *– Hospitals will probably have device reporting systems over and above the usual adverse incident forms.*
- Do you know how to decontaminate a device which needs to be sent for maintenance/repair? *– A necessary but vital chore for the user!*

Information

Manufacturers are required to supply instructions on the medical device, its use and maintenance and they are required to update this as necessary. There should be a copy of this information either with the piece of equipment or nearby on the ward or department. If there are problems with these instructions, this should be reported to your medical engineering department for them to pass on to the manufacturers.

Adverse incidents

When medical devices are used there is the potential for unwanted or unexpected outcomes that affect the safety of patients and others. This may result in an injury to a patient, visitor or member of staff, or breakdown of the devices which means that the patient's treatment is interrupted or compromised, there is misdiagnosis of the patient's condition or the patient's health deteriorates.

Adverse incidents, therefore, must be reported both internally and to the MHRA (Medicines and Healthcare Products Regulatory Agency) using MDA SN (2002/01) and staff should have training in adverse incident reporting.

Hazard notices

The MHRA produces hazard notices, device alerts and safety notices. This is often when they have been contacted about problems from users across the country. You should be notified of these by your medical devices co-ordinator, health and safety manager or similar and it is essential that you follow the instructions in the hazard notice which may include removing the device from use.

Remember what you can do

- Have a working knowledge of the policies for medical devices in your organisation and make sure you follow the key principles.
- Be familiar with the equipment used in your specialty.
- Make sure you are trained to use this equipment.
- Make sure you know how to contact your medical devices co-ordinator (or similar).
- Make sure you train patients and carers who take equipment home.
- Know how to report adverse incidents within the organisation and to the MHRA.
- Act on hazard notices.

References

MDA (2002) Reporting Adverse Incidents and Disseminating Safety Warning. MDA SN 2002/01 MDA, London

Additional reading

Dimond B. (2002) Medical devices regulations and the Medical Devices Agency. *Br J Nursing* **11**(15): 1007–9

MDA (1998) Medical Devices and Equipment Management for Hospital and Community Based Organisations MDA DB 9801. Medical Devices Agency, London + supplement 1 Dec 1999, checks and tests for newly delivered medical devices. London. MDA

Medical Devices Regulations (2002) SI2002 No 618. The Stationery Office, London

NHSE (1999) Controls Assurance in Infection Control: Decontamination of Medical Devices HSC 1999/179

Useful web addresses

www.mhra.gov.uk	Medicines and Healthcare Products Regulatory Agency
www.medical-devices.gov.uk	Specific Medical Devices Section of MHRA
www.dh.gov.uk	Department of Health
www.npsa.nhs.uk	National Patient Safety Agency

Chapter 13

Infection control

Linda Raybould

Hospital-acquired infections are a major problem for the NHS (National Audit Office, 2000). The term 'hospital-acquired' infection has been replaced by 'healthcare-associated' infection (Department of Health, 2002). This is because infections may be transmitted in hospital but more care is now undertaken within the primary care settings exposing patients to the risk of infection.

The significance of healthcare-associated infections has been highlighted by a Department of Health circular (HSC, 2000/02), which urges hospitals to promote high standards of infection control.

National evidence based guidelines for preventing healthcare-associated infections were published in 2001 (Pratt et al, 2001). These standards should be incorporated into nursing practice and be applied by nurses to the care of all hospital in-patients.

Healthcare associated infections

❖ Around 9% of in-patients develop an infection.
❖ Around 5000 patients die annually as a result of these infections.
❖ Infections cost the NHS £1 billion per year.
❖ Hospital patients are susceptible to infection due to age, serious illness, immunosuppression.
❖ Invasive medical treatments increase the likelihood of infection.
❖ The growth of antibiotic resistant organisms
❖ Poor standards of cleanliness.
❖ Pressure on beds leads to higher levels of in-patient hospital moves.

Department of Health, 2002 'Getting Ahead of the Curve'

The Standard principles for preventing hospital-acquired infections are divided into four sections:

- Hospital hygiene.
- Hand decontamination.

- Personal protective clothing.
- Use and disposal of sharps.

Hospital Hygiene

Good hospital hygiene is an integral and important component of a strategy for preventing hospital-acquired infection.

(Pratt et al, 2001).

The NHS Plan (2000) found that patients believed the standards of hospital cleanliness had dropped. Evidence shows that outbreaks of infection are linked to unclean environments (Dancer, 1999). To address this issue the Department of Health has developed 'National Standards of Cleanliness in the NHS' (2003) to improve the quality of the service. Nurses should familiarise themselves with these standards and report any deficiencies.

The environment may also become contaminated if the correct procedures for the handling and disposal of linen and waste are not followed. National guidance is available to address these issues: Hospital Laundry Arrangements (NHSE, 1995) and Health and Safety Executive Safe Disposal of Clinical Waste, 1999).

Hospital hygiene

- ❖ The hospital environment should be visibly clean, free from dust and soilage.
- ❖ Equipment which is used for more than one patient eg commodes should be cleaned in between each patient use.
- ❖ Staff should receive training in the safe handling of used/infected linen and the safe disposal of clinical waste.

Pratt *et al*, 2001

Hand Decontamination

Hands must be decontaminated before and after every episode of patient contact or activity that may result in hands becoming contaminated.

Hands are considered to play a major role in the transmission of infection between patients.

(ICNA, 2002a).

Studies show that nurses do not wash their hands as frequently as they should (Ward et al, 1997). The NMC code of conduct (2004) advises nurses to minimise the risks to patients. All nurses must be responsible for their own hand hygiene. The effectiveness of hand decontamination involves the following:

- risk assessment of the intended activity
- choice of a cleansing agent
- correct hand decontamination technique.

Risk assessment for hand decontamination

To prevent the transfer of micro-organisms wash or apply an alcohol preparation before and after every:

- patient contact
- procedure
- activity that results in potential contamination.

Choice of cleansing agent

Soap and water

In most clinical situations soap and water is sufficient for removing micro-organisms (ICNA, 2002a).

Alcohol-based preparations

Reports indicate that alcohol preparations are more effective in removing bacteria from the hands (Girou et al, 2002). The placement of these products at each patient bedspace has been shown to reduce infection rates (Gopal Rao et al, 2002). However, hands must be visibly clean before use as it is not a cleansing agent. Staff must wash with soap and water after two to three applications of alcohol preparations (ICNA, 2002a).

Aqueous antiseptic solutions

These are handwashing solutions which contain antiseptics such as chlorhexidine, iodophors or triclosan. These products will destroy bacteria on the hands and some will have a residual activity to provide protection against micro-organisms (Pratt et al, 2001).
They are used for:

- aseptic techniques
- caring for vulnerable patients
- caring for patients with transmissible infections.

Hand decontamination techniques

It is essential that nurses cover all aspects of the hands during the decontamination process (Ayliffe et al, 2000).

Hand decontamination

- ❖ Wet hands under running water before applying cleanser.
- ❖ Vigorously rub all surfaces of the hands for 10-15 seconds paying attention to finger tips, thumbs and between the fingers.
- ❖ Rinse hands thoroughly under running water.
- ❖ Dry hands thoroughly on a disposable paper towel.
- ❖ Alcohol rubs/gel are applied to clean dry hands, rubbing hands together until dry.
- ❖ Keep nails short – do not wear artificial nails or nail varnish.
- ❖ Avoid wearing rings, bracelets and wrist watches.
- ❖ Apply hand cream regularly.

Hand Decontamination Guidelines ICNA, 2002a

Personal protective equipment

Nurses should select protective clothing on the basis of a risk assessment of:

- the risk of transmission of micro-organisms to the patient.
- the risk of contamination of the healthcare worker's clothing and skin by the patients blood/body fluids.

Disposable gloves

Healthcare workers wear gloves to:

- prevent the transmission of infection from staff to patients and vice versa
- prevent exposure to blood/body fluids
- prevent exposure to chemicals which may affect the skin.

The use of gloves has increased with the advent of HIV in the 1980s (ICNA, 2002b). Natural rubber latex (NRL) or nitrile gloves are recommended when dealing with blood/body fluids as they offer the best protection against bloodborne viruses (Korniewicz, 2002). Nurses should rationalise their use of NRL gloves as prolonged wearing may lead to latex sensitisation (MDA, 1996). Staff who are concerned about glove reactions should contact the occupational health department. All NRL gloves which are purchased should be low in protein (<50 mg/g), low in chemicals and powder-free.

Staff must undertake a risk assessment to determine the choice of glove for individual tasks.

Non-sterile examination gloves

Latex or synthetic alternative (nitrile)
- ❖ potential exposure to blood/body fluids or synthetic
- ❖ handling sharps
- ❖ handling cytotoxic/disinfectants

Vinyl
- ❖ procedures with low risk of blood/body fluid contamination
- ❖ cleaning with detergent.

Polythene
- ❖ not recommended for clinical use.

Protective Clothing ICNA, 2002c

Disposable aprons

Plastic aprons are worn routinely during clinical activities. Aprons should be worn for one task and then discarded (Pratt et al, 2001).

Disposable plastic aprons

Staff should wear single-use plastic aprons:
* ❖ for potential direct contact with blood/body fluids
* ❖ for direct contact with infectious patients and their environment.

Staff should wear single use, long sleeved impermeable aprons:
* ❖ for situations where there is likely to be extensive contamination.

Protective clothing, ICNA, 2002c

Facial protection

Face masks and eye protection should be worn where there is a risk of blood or body fluids or chemicals, splashing into the face and eyes (Pratt et al, 2001). The types of protection used are:

* goggles
* visors
* face shields (face mask with integral eye protection).

Staff must be provided with equipment that is comfortable to wear and that allows for clear vision (ICNA, 2002c).

Masks for tuberculosis

Masks are worn to protect the wearer from acquiring tuberculosis. The British Thoracic Society (2000) recommend that a dust mist or filtering mask should be worn by staff in certain situations.

Face masks for TB

Staff should wear masks for:
* Suspected or known TB:
  – for cough-inducing procedures – eg bronchoscopy
  – aerosol generating procedures – eg sputum induction
* Suspected/known drug resistant TB (DRTB) or multi-drug resistant TB (MDRTB)

Protective clothing ICNA, 2002c

Safe use and disposal of sharps

The safe handling and disposal of sharps should form part of an overall strategy to protect staff, patients and visitors from bloodborne viruses.

Sharps injuries are regularly reported by healthcare workers (MDA , 2001). These injuries could result in the exposure to serious and potentially fatal bloodborne pathogens such as HIV, hepatitis B and C.

Any healthcare worker who receives a needlestick injury needs to be assessed for the potential risk of infection by a specialist practitioner or occupational health nurse (Pratt et al, 2001).

All sharps injuries are considered preventable (Pratt et al, 2001). The following guidance can help to prevent needlestick injuries:

Sharps disposal

* Dispose of the sharps you use.
* Used sharps must be discarded into a sharps container (UN 3291 and BS 7320) at the point of use.
* Do not pass sharps from hand to hand.
* Needles must not be re-capped.
* Discard needle and syringe as one unit.
* Do not fill sharps containers above the manufacturer's line.
* Needles must not be bent or broken prior to use or disposal.
* Lock the used sharps container when ready for final disposal.

MDA, 2001

Isolation precautions

Patients with transmissible infections are nursed within single rooms to minimise the risk of infection to other patients and staff. The infection control team will provide advice on the appropriate precautions. Each patient should be assessed regularly to determine the need for isolation as the restrictions on their freedom and ability to communicate can be disturbing (Oldman, 1998).

There are two categories of isolation as defined by Philpott-Howard and Casewell, 1994:

Source isolation – to prevent the transfer of micro-organisms from infected patients.

Protective isolation – to protect highly susceptible patients from infection.

Source isolation

This is sub-divided into three sections:

- Strict isolation.
- Standard isolation.
- Blood/body substances isolation.

Strict isolation

This is used for patients with serious but rare infections. These patients should be nursed in specialised infectious diseases units where appropriate facilities are available. The infection control team must be notified if patients with these serious infections are admitted.

Strict isolation

- ❖ Anthrax
- ❖ Diptheria
- ❖ Lassa Fever
- ❖ Plague
- ❖ Rabies
- ❖ Smallpox
- ❖ Viral haemorrhagic fevers

Precautions

❖ Single room – patients not to leave the room without permission.
❖ Gloves and apron for direct contact.
❖ Laundry to be placed into a dissolvable bag and processed as infected.
❖ Filter masks for TB patients.
❖ Non-disposable equipment should be decontaminated. Contact infection control or sterile services department for advice.
❖ Dispose of all waste as clinical waste.

Standard isolation

This is used for patients with infections which may be spread via the air or by direct contact.

Standard isolation

❖ Infections caused by streptococcus pyogenes, eg cellulitis or pharyngitis.
❖ Infections caused by multiple resistant organisms.
❖ Infected dermatitis/eczema/impetigo.
❖ Scabies.
❖ Common infectious diseases eg, chickenpox, shingles, measles, mumps, rubella, whooping cough.
❖ Meningococcal meningitis.
❖ Tuberculosis.

Blood/body substance isolation

These precautions are used when infections may be transmitted by contact with the patient's blood or body fluids.

Blood/body substance isolation

- ❖ Campylobacter
- ❖ Enteric viruses
- ❖ Salmonella
- ❖ Shigella
- ❖ Clostridium difficile
- ❖ Diarrhoea of unknown origin
- ❖ Hepatitis A or E
- ❖ Hepatitis B and C
  Patients with bloodborne viral infections (eg AIDS or HIV or hepatitis B or C) only require isolation if they are bleeding or have a secondary infection. Some of these patients may require a side room for psychological reasons (Ayliffe et al, 2000).

Precautions

- ❖ Single room
- ❖ Gloves and aprons for direct contact with blood/body fluids
- ❖ Laundry to be placed into a dissolvable bag and processed as infected.
- ❖ Non-disposable equipment should be decontaminated. Contact Infection Control or Sterile Services Department for advice.
- ❖ Dispose of all waste as clinical waste.

Protective isolation

This is required to protect susceptible patients from the pathogens within the hospital environment or from infections spread via hospital staff or visitors.

Protective isolation

- ❖ Neutropenia
- ❖ Immunodeficient states
- ❖ Severe dermatitis/burns.

Precautions

- ❖ Single room – visitors with infections should not enter.
- ❖ Gloves and aprons for direct contact and invasive procedures.
- ❖ Waste, laundry, non-disposable equipment should be processed as normal.

Reducing healthcare-related infections

Key requirements

❖ Monitor levels of healthcare-associated infections, eg MRSA clostridium difficile.

❖ Prevent infections associated with catheters, tubes, cannulae and other devices.

❖ Nurses should liaise with bed managers to ensure infected patients are isolated in appropriate facilities.

❖ Clinical teams will demonstrate consistently high stnadards of compliance with infection control procedures, eg hand decontamination, aseptic techniques.

❖ Ensure the prudent use of antibiotics.

❖ Organisations should enure that prevention of infection is a core component of their clinical governance programme.

❖ A national research strategy will be developed to address the gaps in knowledge on how to reduce healthcare-associated infections.

DoH 2003

Remember what you can do

- Take action when the standards of cleanliness in your area fall below an acceptable and safe level.
- To undertake mandatory training that will help you achieve a high standard of infection control.
- Keep up to date with policies on infection control and have a day-to-day working knowledge of these.
- The importance of hand washing in preventing the spread of infection for yourself, other health care professionals, patients and visitors.
- Make sure you and those who work with you wear personal protective clothing and ensure supplies do not run out.
- Make sure you and those who work with you follow the policy and procedure for sharps in order to prevent needlestick injuries.

References

Ayliffe GAJ, Fraise AP, Geddes AM, Mitchell K (2000) Control of Hospital Infection: A Practical Handbook, 4th edition. Arnold, London

British Thoracic Society Guidelines (2000) Control and Prevention of Tuberculosis in the United Kingdom: Code of Practice. *Thorax* **55**: 887–901

Dancer SJ (1999) Mopping up hospital infection. *J Hospital Infection* **43**: 85–100

Department of Health (2000) NHS Plan. The Stationery Office, London

Department of Health (2000). The Management and Control of Hospital Infection. HSC 2000/002, The Stationery Office, London

Department of Health (2002). Getting Ahead of the Curve: A Strategy for Combating Infectious Diseases. The Stationery Office, London

Department of Health (2003). Winning Ways. Report from the Chief Medical Officer. DoH, London

Girou E, Loyeau S, Legrand P et al (2002). Efficacy of handrubbing with alcohol based solution versus standard handwashing with antiseptic soap: randomised clinical trial. *Br Medical J* 325(7360): 362

Gopal Rao G, Jeanes A, Osman M et al (2002). *J Hospital Infection* **50**: 42–7

Health and Safety Executive (1999). Safe Disposal of Clinical Waste: 68. HSE, London

Infection Control Nurses Association (ICNA) (2002a). Hand Decontamination Guidelines. ICNA c/o Fitwise, Bathgate, UK

Infection Control Nurses Association (ICNA) (2002b). A Comprehensive Glove Choice. ICNA c/o Fitwise, Bathgate, UK

Infection Control Nurses Association (ICNA) (2002c). Protective Clothing Principles and Guidance. ICNA c/o Fitwise, Bathgate, UK

Korniewicz DM, Maher El Masri MS, Broyles JM et al (2002) Peformance of latex and non-latex medical examination gloves during simulated use. *Am J Infection Control* **30**: 133–8

Medical Devices Agency (MDA) (1996). Latex Sensitisation in the Healthcare Setting. Use of Latex Gloves (DB(96)01). The Stationery Office, London.

Medical Devices Agency (MDA) (2001). Safe Use and Disposal of Sharps. MDA SN 2001 (19). MDA, London

National Audit Office (2000). The Management and Control of Hospital Infection in Acute NHS Trusts in England. HC230 Session 1999-00: National Audit Office, London.

National Health Service Executive (NHSE) (1995). Hospital Laundry Arrangements for Used and Infected Linen. HSG (95) 18:4. NHSE, Leeds.

NHS Estates (2003). National Standards of Cleanliness in the NHS. NHS Estates, The Stationery Office, London.

Nursing and Midwifery Council (NMC) (2004). Code of Professional Conduct. NMC, London

Oldman, T. (1998) Isolated cases. *Nurs Times* **94**(11) (Supplement)

Philpott-Howard J and Casewell M (1994). Hospital Infection Control, Policies and Practical Procedures. London, Bailliere Tindall.

Pratt RJ, Pellowe C, Loveday HP, Robinson N, Smith GW and the epic guideline development team (2001). The epic project: developing national evidence-based guidelines for preventing healthcare sssociated infections. *J Hospital Infection* **47** (supplement) 521–37.

Ward V, Wilson J, Taylor L, Cookson B and Glynn A (1997). Preventing Hospital Acquired Infection. Clinical Guidelines. Public Health Laboratory Service, London.

Additional reading

Carol M et al (2002) Assessment of hand washing practices with chemical and microbiological methods: preliminary results from a prospective cross over study. *Am J Infection Control* **30**(6) October: 334–40

DoH (2001) Standard principles for preventing hospital acquired infections. *J Hospital Infection* **47**(Supplement) S21—S37

DoH (2001) Agenda for clinical governance. *J Hospital Infection* **47** (Supplement)

NHS Estates (2002) Infection Control in the Built Environment. NHS Estates Executive organisation of the DOH

Plowman R et al (2000) Socioeconomic Burden of Hospital Acquired Infection .Public Health Laboratory Service: London

Useful websites

www.cleanhospitals.com	Clean hospitals programme
www.dh.gov.uk	Department of Health
www.icna.co.uk	The Infection Control Nurses Association
www.med.virginia.edu/epinet	Exposure prevention information network (EPINET)
www.nhsestates.gov.uk	NHS estates
www.phls.co.uk	Public Health Laboratory Service
www.epic.tvu.ac.uk	Epic initiative contributes to the evidence base for infection control practice, Thames Valley University
www.needlestickforum.com	Needlestick forum

Useful Addresses

Fitwise, Drumcross Hall, Bathgate, EH48 4JT. Tel: 01506 811077. Email: info@fitwise.co.uk

Chapter 14

Assessing and managing the patient's environment

Jeanette Welsh

In the previous three chapters the legislation and regulations concerning many aspects of the patients' environment have been covered. This chapter will focus on how the environment should be assessed and managed to ensure it meets the legislation and is safe and secure for patients and visitors and that it is an appropriate working environment for staff.

Providing a comfortable environment

Health and Safety regulations require that sufficient light, heat, space and ventilation are provided. Neither patients nor staff should find the environment unbearably hot or too cold and there should be adequate space for beds, lockers, equipment, stores, IT equipment and offices.

In developing the NHS Plan, the Government (DoH, 2000) undertook a widespread public consultation exercise which showed that patients wanted hospitals to be clean, tidy, safe and welcoming. As a result the Clean Hospitals Environment Programme was set up (NHS Estates, 2001). This seeks to ensure hospitals' standards of cleanliness and tidiness are being maintained and improved. The programme is closely linked with improving infection control.

Keeping wards and departments tidy will help to remove environmental hazards for patients and prevent injury. To ensure the area you work in is kept tidy, safe and welcoming you should ensure:

- The temperature is comfortable for patients and staff. You may need to check with patients as they may be reluctant to 'cause a fuss'. You should know how to contact the heating engineer both during and outside normal working hours. You should also know how to obtain blankets and fans.
- Any equipment not being used is kept stored.
- Any trailing flexes and leads are removed or protected.
- Spilt liquids are dealt with immediately by putting hazard warnings in place and call appropriate personnel to deal with the hazard.
- Newly mopped floors have a warning cone.

- Clutter, such as chairs left after visiting, abandoned trolleys or other pieces of equipment, are removed and stored.
- Overflowing rubbish bins are emptied.
- There are warning notices on water boilers in kitchen areas.
- Condemned equipment is disposed of according to your local policy.
- Areas restricted to staff are clearly marked and doors kept closed when possible.

Easy Access

The Disability Discrimination Act (1995) requires that the hospital is easily accessible for all people with disabilities. This does not just mean physical access; it also covers signage being clear for those who have a visual impairment. It also means providing hearing loops in consultation areas and other communication aids for those who are hard of hearing.

Within your working environment you should:

- ensure that there are no obstructions for people with mobility problems as described above
- make arrangements so that patients and visitors who have specially trained dogs for support can continue to use them
- make arrangements with patients to bring in and use their normal mobility aids while in hospital
- discuss with patients how they want to communicate their disability with others, for example some magnetic symbols can be used discretely on bed ends if patients wish
- ensure you know how to use any communication aids
- ensure you and others are aware of any patients with disabilities and what they will find helpful in minimising risks from such disabilities

Infection control regulations

These regulations require that everything possible is done to minimise the transmission of infection from one patient to another and prevent hospital-acquired infection. Illness reduces a patient's ability to fight infection and so all areas have to be kept much cleaner than most people would keep their homes.

To improve the control of infection in your environment you should look for and take action when:

- dust is found under and behind furniture
- dried blood or other secretions are found on the floor, on cot sides of beds or trolleys or on wires of monitoring equipment
- used bedpans, vomit bowls and urine bottles are left sitting on lockers, bedside tables or in the sluice
- mops are left in buckets of dirty water
- discarded, used wound dressings are found
- bedside lockers and tables become cluttered
- sharps boxes are full and overflowing
- furniture is soiled or stained
- you see clinical staff not washing their hands after procedures or between patients.

You should ensure that:

- hand gel is available at ward entrances and in ward areas
- gloves are provided in the clinical area
- antiseptic handwashing solutions with pump-action dispensers are used
- taps with 'elbow' handles, that allow staff to switch them off with elbows rather than freshly washed hands, are used
- there are clear notices to patients on infection control eg not to swap footstools round, not to share blankets or pillows and to wash their hands after using the toilet
- you know how to contact domestic cleaning services to do urgent cleaning jobs
- you keep the ward sister/charge nurse informed when problems with cleanliness and infection control persist.

Hazardous substances in the workplace

The COSHH (Control of Substances Hazardous to Health, 1994) regulations referred to in chapter 11 require that certain safeguards are put in place in the working environment. There should be a written document in each clinical area covering the chemicals and other hazardous substances used in that area, giving the risks to health and what should be done to minimise these risks. You should know where these risk assessments and safe systems of work are kept and be aware of your responsibilities when using these substances. Ensure:

- drugs are locked away
- lotion cupboards are also kept locked when not in use
- cleaning solutions are clearly labelled in the sluice, cleaners' store and kitchen and are appropriately stored

There has been particular concern regarding the use of gluteraldehyde (Cidex) in the cleaning of endoscopes and surgical instruments, which can cause asthma-type symptoms. The use of gluteraldehyde is now very tightly controlled. You should be aware of the controls within your hospital and your responsibilities and also the action required if there is any spillage of this substance.

Manual handling

The importance of safe manual handling has been highlighted in chapter 11 along with the potential consequences of poor manual handling. You should consider the following which will help prevent injury to yourself and others.

1. Your organisation should have a policy for manual handling and should provide training with regular updates. You should have training to enable you to use equipment safely and ensure you are updated on new techniques.
2. You should also know how to undertake a risk assessment for manual handling individual patients.
3. In the clinical environment you should ensure:
- adequate space around beds for hoists and manoeuvring
- adequate space in bathrooms for bath hoists and accessing patients
- adequate storage facilities for hoists and other manual handling devices
- there are dust and stain free slide sheets
- manual handling devices appropriate to the clinical speciality are available (eg Immoturn in orthopaedic areas, Stryker frames in spinal injury units)
- no staff under eighteen undertake manual handling
- no pregnant or nursing mothers (until baby is one year old) lift from floor level, even as part of a team
- staff lifting boxes etc do so in two moves from floor level
- hoists and other devices are marked with their weight limit
- hoists are clearly labelled with inspection dates (every six months) and service dates (every year)

- no member of staff ever takes all or a substantial part of a patient's weight (except babies and small children)
- faulty or damaged equipment is taken out of service immediately and repaired or condemned.
- all members of staff demonstrate in their work the five principles of manual handling:
    - spine in line
    - stable base
    - soft knees
    - held loads close to their bodies
    - looking in the direction they want to go.
- there are beds and trolleys that can be varied in height to enable patients to get out of bed easily or sit themselves up without nursing assistance
- monkey poles are available on beds in areas where patients are unable to use their legs fully (eg. orthopaedics, vascular surgery)
- IT equipment is ergonomically positioned
- chairs are available that support backs well at nursing stations, in dayrooms, in interview rooms
- there is a lack of clutter

Preventing harm

'First do no harm' – is enshrined in the Hippocratic oath. Staying in hospital can give rise to a number of complications but action can be taken to reduce the risk of these developing.

The development of pressure sores

These are otherwise known as bedsores or decubitus ulcers. Details of patient management can be found in *Chapter 7* but in the clinical environment you should ensure:

- there are pressure relieving mattresses
- there are pressure relieving cushions in wheelchairs
- that patient risk assessments are completed for each patient
- that pillows are placed so that patients' heels are suspended not put under pressure
- patient comfort rounds are undertaken regularly (*Chapter 4*)

- that patients are encouraged to get up and move around regularly.

Deep vein thrombosis and chest infections

These complications arise when patients remain inactive in bed or in a chair. You should ensure:

- patients are being encouraged to move around regularly
- an anticoagulation screen is done for all long-stay patients
- inpatient anticoagulation is considered for all long-stay patients
- anti-embolic stockings are fitted to all long-stay and surgical patients
- where patients are unable to get out of bed that they have regular chest physiotherapy and are repositioned at two-hourly intervals
- patients are actively encouraged to exercise in bed
- regular passive exercises are carried out in unconscious or paralysed patients .

Preventing falls

Accidental falls within a hospital setting are a major cause of concern and have become a priority area. Falls are a major cause of disability, may delay discharge, lead to complications and require additional treatment as well as causing unnecessary suffering.

All staff should be able to reduce factors which result in falls and understand their responsibilities in the event of a patient falling. These include:

- Reducing environmental factors such as:
  - ensuring the call bell is within easy reach
  - ensuring brakes on equipment are in working order and are used
  - maintaining a tidy environment.
- Being able to undertake an assessment of a patient's risk of falling while in hospital and plan appropriate interventions to minimise the risk.
- Using bed rails only when necessary and ensuring they are in working order.
- Keeping beds in lowered positions or putting the mattress on the floor.
- Using pressure alarm systems.
- Informing medical staff immediately and family at the earliest opportunity of falls and following prescribed treatment plan.
- Ensuring patients and relatives are provided with information on fall prevention.

Equipment and medical devices

Resuscitation equipment should be easily available in all clinical areas. The management of cardiopulmonary resuscitation events are covered in chapter 6. However, equipment should be checked and maintained to ensure it is readily available in the clinical area. You should ensure there are:

- daily checks on defibrillators
- checks on contents of resuscitation trolley/backpack daily and after every use
- you are updated in basic life support techniques annually as a minimum.

Medical devices are used in all clinical areas and are subject to the regulations of the Medical Devices Agency and must comply with several standards. These regulations are highlighted in Chapter 12 along with requirements for reporting incidents. A large number of critical incidents are traced back to misuse of medical devices and it is therefore essential that safeguards are put in place in hospitals. These include:

- All medical devices being selected by a purchasing group within the organisation.
- All medical devices having a maintenance schedule, undertaken and monitored by medical engineering staff.
- All nursing staff being trained to use every medical device in their clinical area and being updated as necessary.
- Records of such training held at ward/department level and trust level.
- Patient and relatives being taught how to use devices as appropriate.

You should ensure:

- you are aware of your local policy for medical devices and are able to comply with it
- you have been trained in the use of all devices you are expected to use in your work
- faulty equipment is labelled and taken out of use and appropriately labelled
- maintenance request books are available and requests are promptly attended to
- notes on medical devices equipment should show the last dates of calibration and servicing
- you check the safety of each device or piece of equipment before you use it.

Violence and aggression

Prevention is better than cure. Many hospitals are implementing zero tolerance measures to violence and aggression. Ensure:

- You know the policy and procedures for handling violence and aggression in your organisation.
- You are able to recognise the early warning signs such as, restlessness, raised voice, changes in behaviour and facial expression, pacing up and down and unpredictable movements.
- You are able to apply some general preventative measures such as:
  - keeping patients and their relatives informed of treatment and progress and being willing to answer questions
  - greeting relatives in an open and relaxed manner
  - ensuring you body language and tone of voice is open rather than defensive
  - providing a quiet area.
- There are locks on restricted areas.
- Panic buttons are available in staff-only areas.
- You are aware of procedures to summon help.

This chapter has highlighted several points that should be considered when assessing the clinical environment.

Remember

- ❖ If you are not safe, your patients are not safe and you have been entrusted with their safety.
- ❖ The environment is important to patients and makes a significant contribution to the outcomes of care.

Remember what you can do

- Be constantly on the look out for environmental hazards and take action to minimise the effects.
- To keep up to date with policies relating to the environment and have a day-to-day working knowledge of these.
- If there are problems with aspects of the environment that are out of your control, make sure your line manager is aware of them.

- Undertake mandatory training that will help you maintain a safe and pleasant environment for patients.
- Make sure the equipment you use is right for the job and is in good working order before you use it.
- Remember you have a legal responsibility in relation to the health and safety of others.

References

Department of Health (2000) NHS Plan. The Stationery Office, London

Disability Discrimination Act (2005)

NHS Estates (2001) National Standards of Cleanliness for NHS. NHS Estates Executive Organisation of the DOH, London

Additional reading

Beech B (2001) Zero Tolerance of violence against health care staff. *Nurs Standard* **15**(16): 39–41

Brennan W (1998) Aggression and Violence examining the theories. *Nurs Standard* **12**(27): 36–7

Department of Health (1999) NHS Zero Tolerance Zone. We Don't Have to Take This. Resource Pack. The Stationery Office, London

Department of Health (2000) The Management and Control of Hospital Infection. HSC 2000/002. The Stationery Office, London

Duxbury J (2003) Testing a new tool: the management of aggression and violence attitude scale (MAVAS) *Nurs Res* **10**(4): 39–52

Garnham P (2001) Understanding and dealing with anger aggression and violence. *Nurs Standard* **16**(6): 37–42, 44–5

Medical Devices Agency (2000) Equipped to Care: The Safe Use of Medical Devices in the 21st Century. MDA, London

Well J, Bowes L (2002) How prevalent is violence toward nurses in general hospitals in the UK. *J Adv Nurs* **39**(3): 230–40

Useful web sites

www.hse.gov.uk/healthsevices   Health and Safety Executive

www.dh.gov.uk   Department of Health
www.medical-devices.gov.uk   Medical Devices
www.nmc-uk.org   Nursing and Midwifery Council

Section 3
Clinical quality

Clinical quality and its increasing importance

The expectations of patients and members of the public regarding the quality of health care have risen dramatically over the last two decades as a result of the rise of consumerism. From the users point of view the health service was seen as being geared to the needs and convenience of those who ran it and worked in it. Consumer power has increased during the last 30 years resulting in some changes as users are increasingly challenging the decision making processes of health professionals and managers.

The Community Health Councils (CHC) set up in the 1970s enabled the public to demand a say in how local health services were organised as there was a requirement for Health Authorities to consult with them when any major change or redistribution of service were planned, such as the closure of hospitals. They also had a right to visit NHS premises to monitor quality and provision of services. Although CHCs are now disbanded (since December 2003) many of their roles have been taken over by Patient and Public Involvement Forums which are designed to ensure an even greater involvement of the public in the planning, development and monitoring of standards in health services.

The various Governments of the last three decades have also played their part in involving patients and the public more. In the 1990s with the Patients Charter (DoH 1991) the rights of patients to access health care was set out and this served to raise expectations. In developing its plans for reforming the health service in the late 1990s the labour government actively consulted with a wide representation of the population and although there are differing views there was much consensus on areas where quality needed to be improved. These included, quicker access to health care, improved standards of cleanliness and hygiene, need to reduce infections, particularly in hospitals, need for better information and more choice, the need for more doctors and nurses and the need to know who was 'in charge'.

There has also been an increase in the so called compensation culture which is proving increasingly costly for the NHS. It is important that as much as possible is done to ensure that care is done in the right way, the first time to reduce the risk of claims and ensure patients early recovery.

These factors have resulted in the introduction of many initiatives designed to improve the quality of care and these are described in the chapters in this section.

Chapter 15 Clinical Quality provides an overview of the clinical governance framework which is being used through out the NHS to improve quality through introducing clinical effective practices, auditing, managing risks effectively, using information for making effective clinical decisions, developing and managing staff effectively and having good strategic leadership and sound management to support this. *Chapter 16 Standards of Care* highlights the influence that government, professional and statutory bodies have on standards of care and how these are implemented at a local level. It also includes the role of the Matron and the Patients and Public Involvement Forums in improving and maintaining standards. *Chapter 17 Expanding Professional Practice* describes how there is increased access to and improved standards of care for patients as a result of nurses expanding and extending their roles. *Chapter 18 Research and evidence based nursing* provides an introduction to the main issues and relevance to nurses of research and describes the value of nursing research and evidence in underpinning practice. *Chapter 19 Clinical Information* describes how information is used to support nurses in the organisation, management and delivery of care, in employing and managing staff and in managing performance.

References

DoH (1991) The Patient's Charter. Department of Health, London

Chapter 15

Clinical quality

Derek Eaves

There is an old saying: 'beauty is in the eye of the beholder'. To a certain extent the same can be said about the quality of care given to a patient. One's perception of 'quality' will depend on a number of factors including knowledge base, previous experience and the part of the world in which you live. So, to a certain extent, any assessment of quality will be subjective.

However, from a number of sources such as professional bodies, specialist university departments and national agencies, there is a growing body of evidence on what is a 'good' or acceptable standard of care in the United Kingdom.

One of the aims of the latest government initiative on quality is to bring all this evidence together from the many disparate sources. This initiative is called clinical governance and this was first described in A First Class Service (DoH, 1998). Although there is much technical jargon around related to clinical governance, Lilley (1999) got it right when he said it is 'doing anything and everything required to maximise quality'.

The aims of clinical governance

- the continuous improvement of patients' services and care
- a patient-centred approach
- a commitment to quality
- up-to-date professional practice and good supervision
- reduction of risk from clinical errors and adverse events, to learn from mistakes.

Clinical governance framework

While the above guidelines are good as a starting point, it is useful to have a specific framework, which one can use to ensure that clinical governance is happening in your area of work. Clinical Governance can be seen to be made up of a number of elements (Figure 15.1)

Figure 15.1: The elements of clinical governance

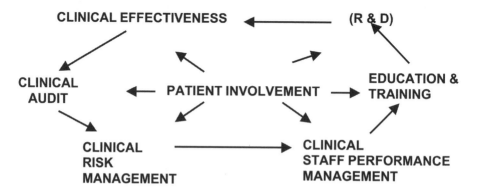

It is worth discussing these elements in turn, although some will be in more detail than others, as the latter are covered in other chapters of this book.

Clinical effectiveness

Nurses, like all professionals, aim to give the most appropriate care and treatment to patients. However, how do you know if you are doing this? As stated above, there is a considerable amount of evidence now available on what is the most appropriate drug, technique, care process or intervention for a particular condition or illness. Staff within the various specialities need to draw up explicit statements about appropriate care and treatment processes. These statements are given a variety of titles, some of which are:

- clinical guidelines or protocols
- integrated care pathways
- standards of care.

These can be multidisciplinary, for example the nursing and medical care that all patients with a myocardial infarction should be given, or uni-professional, for example the nursing care of all patients with a urinary catheter. In other words, the teams looking after a particular group of patients have decided on what it is they are trying to provide and achieve. These statements should be based on the latest research evidence and expert opinion which is available from such sources as:

- National Institute for Health and Clinical Excellence (NICE)
- National Service Frameworks – NSFs
- Professional Bodies (eg. Royal College of Nursing)
- National Electronic Library for Health (NELH).

Clinical audit

Once you and your team have guidelines and standards you can then start to undertake audit. Audit is checking whether you are actually achieving the standards you have set or following the guidelines you have drawn up. It is likely that you are not reaching 100% of what you have set out to achieve all of the time. This may be for a variety of reasons, such as staff not always being aware of the guidelines in the first place, poor communication or teamwork, or issues to do with resources. After undertaking audit, the team should be sitting down and reflecting on the results and deciding how they can improve their performance.

As well as self- and internally-generated clinical audit, clinicians and trusts are also subject to audit by outside organisations and bodies. The Commission for Health Improvement (CHI, 2002) was set up to undertake this role. Each trust was initially assessed every three to four years on its clinical governance arrangements. A report was published and the trust had to draw up an action plan based on the results of the assessment. Both the reports and action plans from all trusts are available on its website at www.healthcarecommision.org. uk. From 2005 each trust is sbject to an Annual Health Check instead. It should be remembered that this organisation has other roles too, such as investigating specific major incidents. Its role of monitoring clinical quality increased further in 2004 when its designation changed to the Healthcare Commission.

Clinical risk management

The results of a clinical audit may show you are not reaching 100% of the standard all of the time and risks to patients may be identified. It is important that these and all risks are managed in a systematic way. Nurses should become involved in at least the following three risk management activities:

Risk assessments

Each trust will have a policy on risk assessments, which are undertaken both as a preventative measure, for example with each specialty/ward considering the main risks to patients and how they can be reduced, and as a follow-up procedure after an incident or complaint to prevent a re-occurrence. As part of this process, nurses will have to consider undertaking risk assessments on a wide range of issues such as communication, team working, staffing and medical devices. The trust is required to draw up a register of risks so that resources and actions can be directed at the more important ones.

Adverse incident reporting

In general, there is a good culture within nursing to report when adverse incidents occur, whether it is a patient fall, minor drug administration errors or major events which have a serious effect on the patient. Unfortunately, in the past there has been a 'blame' culture in the NHS, which has meant that any nurse involved in a drug error has automatically been taken through the disciplinary process. This is now changing with the realisation that many incidents are mainly the result of 'systems' failures rather than individual clinician error alone. In other words, the underlying organisational and team factors, for example, issues related to induction, training, teamwork, packaging and storage, need to be identified by thorough investigation. It is only when these factors are brought to light through what is termed root cause analysis that changes can be made to prevent such errors recurring. The National Patient Safety Agency, a centralized body which has one aim of sharing the needed changes across the country.

Achieving CNST standards

Thirdly, nurses should be aware that their hospital is a member of the Clinical Negligence Scheme for Trusts (CNST). This means that the hospital has to follow a number of risk management standards some of which have implications for nurses. For instance, as well as undertaking risk assessments and reporting incidents, nurses should have regular updates on such topics as cardiopulmonary resuscitation, blood transfusion protocols and handwashing techniques. In addition, nurses should be involved in regular auditing of care records. Always remember the 10 golden rules of risk management:

- Act within your own competence.
- Do no harm.
- Follow policies and guidelines.
- Report adverse incidents and 'near misses'.
- Obtain informed consent from patients.
- Write full and legible notes.
- Maintain confidentiality.
- Learn from mistakes.
- Ask if you are unsure.
- Report any concerns about poor practice.

Staff performance management

It is essential for good clinical quality that all staff are competent in their roles. Each ward should have a regular system of appraisal for all its staff. All nurses should be sitting down with a senior member of staff at least yearly when an assessment of performance is undertaken and job objectives for the forthcoming year can be agreed. It is also an opportunity for the member of staff to raise any issues of concern. From the assessment, a personal development plan should also be agreed in which areas for training and development over the next 12 months are identified.

Nurses should also be aware that, as well as taking responsibility for their own competence, they also have some responsibility for the competence of their colleagues. In other words, if they have concerns about a colleague's competence or behaviour they have a duty to report this. Each hospital will have a whistleblowing policy regarding this.

Education and training

Having well-trained and educated staff is key to ensuring clinical quality. This begins with pre-registration training. You and your colleagues can do much to encourage a positive and stimulating learning environment for student nurses. Of particular importance are:

- encouraging a questioning and inquiring approach in students
- ensuring they have a mentor or supervisor who will work with them for much of their placement

- ensuring their learning needs and progress are discussed with them throughout their placement
- providing them with a range of opportunities to see what happens to patients both on and off the ward or department
- ensuring they have the opportunity to shadow other health care professionals
- ensuring there is good liaison between your area and the education link teachers in the educational provider
- ensuring they have access to information and discuss aspects of care with them to link theory and practice.

It is also important to keep professional and clinical practice up to date for qualified nurses and pointers to assist you in this are included in *Chapters 23* and *24.*

Research and development (R&D)

While it is not necessary for every nurse to be an expert researcher, every nurse should be aware of the latest research on the care processes they are involved with. This means that all nurses should be providing evidence based care or clinically effective care, as discussed above. Research and development are covered in more detail in *Chapter 18.*

Patient and public involvement

The role of patients and the public is becoming increasingly important in developing clinical quality. The Commission for Patient and Public Involvement in Health was established early in 2003 to champion and promote involvement of the public in decisions that affect their health. It has the responsibility for overseeing the structures to involve people in planning, developing, monitoring and evaluating health services. These include:

The Patient Advice and Liaison Service (PALS) – advises patients families and carers, provides information on NHS services, listens to concerns and helps sort out problems quickly. Each trust will have a PALS. (*Chapter 5* for more information)

The Patient and Public Involvement Forum – intended to independently watch over the quality of local healthcare, find out what people really think, influence local and national decisions which impact on health. Forums have been set up since December 2003 (*Chapter 16*).

The Independent Complaints Advocacy Service (ICAS) – has been set up to help individuals pursue complaints and ensure they have access to the support they need to articulate their concerns.

Contact for PALS and ICAS are available in each trust.

Clinical governance should ensure that the patient's perspective is taken into consideration in all elements of healthcare. This includes patients being involved in policy decisions when new services are being discussed at organisational level and the individual patient being involved in evaluating and monitoring care at ward level. There should be a range of different ways that feedback is obtained from patients: through surveys, comment cards, suggestions schemes and other similar mechanisms.

To be fully involved in decisions about healthcare, patients need to have information. This ranges from having information on what services and standards they can expect, to having information about their condition and treatment so that they can make informed choices and consent to treatment in the full knowledge of what the options, risks and consequences are for them.

Use of information

Information is essential to support clinical governance and improve the quality of care. There should be good information management systems which enable you to have access to policies, procedures, guidelines and standards that will guide your practice. You should also have access to information to monitor performance and outcomes of care so that you can make improvements. There should also be policies and processes that ensure confidentiality of information about patients and staff. More information on this can be found in *chapter 19*.

Importance of teamworking

Lastly, it has to be remembered that, while all of the above processes will depend on the competence and motivation of each individual practitioner they are also influenced by how well the team works together. Each professional does not work in isolation. Not only does the ward team of nurses need to work well to provide good quality care, but so does the wider multidisciplinary team. Both the nursing team and the multidisciplinary team need to regularly meet and reflect on clinical quality and prioritise on the best ways of improving care.

Using the framework above, the team should be drawing up guidelines and protocols, agreeing which audits to undertake, assessing risks and monitoring incidents, complaints and the results of patient feedback in order to agree an action plan. This is clinical governance in action.

Remember what you can do

- Use evidence based guidelines and standards in your practice.
- Keep up to date with research and best practice for your specialty
- Learn how to access evidence through the internet, journals, books and other resources.
- Seek help from your clinical audit department to check you are achieving the required standards in your area.
- Report any risks you identify.
- Ensure you know how to report any incidents.
- Keep up to date with the risks identified in your area and take the agreed action to minimize these.
- Implement the 10 golden rules of risk management.
- Contribute to your area becoming a positive learning environment.
- Consider how you can involve patients more in their care and treatment.
- Consider how you can use information to improve care in your area.

References

Commission for Health Improvement (2002) A Guide to Clinical Governance Reviews – A Resource Book to Support the Clinical Governance Reviewer Training Course. CHI, London

DoH (1998) A First Class Service: Quality in the New NHS. DoH, London

Lilley (1999) Making Sense of Cinical Governance. Radcliffe Medical Press, Abingdon

Additional Reading

Bishop V, Scott I (eds) (2000) Challenges in Clinical Practice – Professional Development in Nursing. Palgrave, Basingstoke

Bradley L, Rees C (2003) Reducing nutritional risk in hospital: the red tray. *Nurs Standard* **17**(26): 33–7

Currie L (2002) The nursing view of Clinical Governance. *Nurs Standard* **16**(27): 40–4

Dimond B (2002) Whistle-blowing and the Public Interest Disclosure Act 1998. *Br J Nurs* **11**(20): 1307–9

Field A, Reid B (2002) An analysis of an audit tool of ward-based practice. *Nurs Standard* **16**(40): 37–9

Lawton S, Wimpenny P (2003) Continuing professional development : a review. *Nurs Standard* **17**(24): 41–4

Lugon M, Secker Walker J (2002) Clinical Governance: Making it Happen. Royal Society of Medicine Press

McSherry R et al (2001) Clinical Governance: A Guide to Implementation for Health Care Professionals. Blackwell Scientific, Oxford

Weston A, Chamber R, Boath E (2001) Clinical Effectiveness and Clinical Governance for Midwives. Radcliffe, Oxford

Useful web pages

www.nice.org.uk	National Institute for Health and Clinical Excellence
www.healthcommission.org.uk	Healthcare Commission
www.nelh.nhs.uk	National Electronic Library for Health
www.rcn.org.uk	Royal College of Nursing
www.cppih.org	Commission for patient and public involvement
www.nursing-standard.co.uk	Nursing Standard
www,dh.gov.uk	Department of Health
www,npsa.nhs.uk	National Patient Safety Agency
www,modern.nhs.uk	NHS Modernisation Agency

Chapter 16

Standards of care

Ann Close

Concerns about standards of care or service are often expressed anecdotally and are often picked up by the press and made into a big news story, locally or nationally. There are many examples of this over recent years, for example patients requiring intensive care having to be transported for hundreds of miles to find a bed, patients waiting for many hours on trolleys in hospital corridors or stories about hospitals being dirty and reservoirs for the spread of infection. Episodes such as these have led governments, statutory bodies, and managers to review practices and make changes to improve the standards provided for patients. This chapter looks at how the government and professional and regulatory bodies can influence standards and how standards can be used locally to improve nursing care. In addition, the role of the matron and patient and public involvement forums in maintaining standards is discussed.

National standards

The Government's influence

Since the beginning of the 1990s successive governments have put various plans in place to improve the quality and standards of care provided for patients. In the early 1990s the NHS and Community Care Act (1990) came into force with the aim of raising the standard of health and health care and improving the efficiency and effectiveness of the health service through creating internal markets, providing better management which involved more clinicians, through devolved decision making and placing greater emphasis on information giving and health promotion.

With the change of government towards the end of the 1990s, plans to reform and modernise the NHS were set out in *The NHS Plan – a plan for investment, a plan for reform.* (DoH 2000). This plan recognised that there had been a lack of national standards and, as a result, a number of actions have been taken to change this.

In February 2004 the Department of Health began consultation on proposals for introducing a series of key standards for the quality of care across the NHS in England. (DoH, 2004). The purpose of these standards is 'to provide the foundations for a common high quality of healthcare throughout England and to clarify what the NHS can and should be reaching for in its ambitions both for the public and for healthcare professionals.' There are twenty-four core and ten developmental standards. The core standards are intended to establish a level of quality care which can be expected by all NHS patients and include such things as 'patients must be able to access emergency care promptly' and hospitals and surgeries should be safe and secure and meet national levels of cleanliness. The developmental standards are designed to enable the overall quality of care to rise as additional resources are invested and new developments are introduced. All NHS organisations are required to make a public declaration on the extent to which they meet the core standards in April 2006. Monitoring of standards will be undertaken by the Healthcare Commission annually in an 'annual Healthcheck' (Healthcare Commission, 2005).

Patients' Charters

In 1991 the Government launched the *Patient's Charter* (DoH, 1991) and for the first time national rights and standards were made explicit. The charter set out the standards of what patients can expect from the National Health Service in relation to access to services including their health records, waiting time for treatment, rights to information and rights to have a named qualified nurse responsible for their care. There have been subsequent additions in the form of the *Maternity Charter* (DoH, 1994) and the *Children's Charter* (DoH 1996)and an update entitled *The Patient's Charter and You* (DoH, 1995).

These charters did have a considerable impact on the service. Patients and the public are more aware of their rights and there have been improvements to services including waiting times for treatment and for admission to hospital and quicker access to care. There was, however, a more negative impact in that, although patients were aware of their rights these are sometimes perceived as unrealistic by healthcare professionals who felt that patients do not recognise their responsibilities for their healthcare. The balance between rights and responsibilities has been addressed to a certain extent in a later update – *Your Guide to the NHS* (DoH, 2001a) but this later version has a different emphasis and does not seem to have had as much influence or impact as the initial charter.

National Service Frameworks

The Department of Health led work to establish national standards which are set out in a series of *National Service Frameworks* (NSF) (HSC, 1998). The aim of each NSF is to set national standards and define service models and each will include an assessment of the health and social care needs to be addressed, the evidence of effective and efficient interventions and organisational arrangements, the present position regarding the service, the issues to be tackled and the resource implications. To date, a number of NSFs have been produced including *Coronary Heart Disease, Mental Health, Older People, Renal, Diabetes* and *Paediatrics*. In order to assist with implementation the standards are underpinned by clear statements of the evidence base and these are disseminated through clinical guidelines. A set of performance measures are included to check on the extent of implementation. Details of the NSF can be accessed through the Department of Health website.

National Institute of Clinical Excellence

Prior to 1999 there were frequent complaints that access to expensive medicines depended on where the individual lived and this was often referred to as the 'post code lottery'. Also best practice was slow at filtering through systems to be implemented across the NHS. As a result The National Institute of Clinical Excellence (NICE) was established in 1999. Its aim is to ensure uniformly high standards are spread across the NHS. NICE gives advice on the clinical and cost effectiveness of new and existing health technologies including medicines, diagnostic tests and surgical procedures. By identifying which new developments most improve patient care, NICE helps to spread new treatments of good value quickly across the NHS and protects patients from outdated and inefficient treatment. Since January 2002 organisations have had three months from the date of publication to implement the guidance (see website address).

Essence of Care

The NHS Plan (2000) highlighted the importance of the fundamental and basic aspects of care and of improving the patients' experience. *The Essence of Care* was launched in February 2001 (DoH, 2001b) to provide practitioners for all professional groups with a tool to help them take a patient-focused and structured approach to sharing and comparing practice. The tool requires health care professionals to work with patients to identify best practice and to develop action plans to improve care.

Patients, carers and professionals worked together to agree and describe good quality care and best practice. This resulted in bench marks covering eight areas:

- continence and bladder and bowel care
- personal and oral hygiene
- food and nutrition
- pressure ulcers
- privacy and dignity
- record keeping
- safety of clients with mental health needs in acute mental health and general hospital settings
- principles of self care

From July 2002 further work was done to add a ninth area focusing on communication between patients, and/or carers and healthcare professionals. All the sets of benchmarks are interrelated and complement each other (Modernisation Agency, 2003).

Essence of Care benchmarking is a process of comparing, sharing and developing practice in order to achieve and sustain best practice. Changes and improvements focus on the indicators since these are items that patients, carers and professionals believed were important in achieving the benchmarks of best practice. The stages involved are:

1. To agree best practice.
2. To assess clinical areas against best practice.
3. To produce and implement an action plan aimed at achieving best practice.
4. To disseminate improvement and or review the action plan.

Essence of Care encourages changes and improvements in care which can be local to a ward or department or can be carried across an organisation. For example, nurses working in an ITU on the privacy and dignity standard were concerned that patients were not wearing nightwear. Although they understood the reason for this – that the traditional gowns restricted access to the lines and equipment – they felt that patient's dignity was compromised. As a result, the staff worked with the sewing room to design tabards especially for the purpose and have worked with some patient groups to fund this. Staff across a trust have implemented a 'curtain peepers' code which requires all staff to ask before entering screen areas around beds and trolleys.

Most trusts have identified a structure and processes to implement *Essence of Care*. You should find out how this operates in your organisation. If there is no process then you should discuss this with your senior nursing colleagues.

Other standards

The Department of Health issues guidance on a wide range of topics such as infection control, medical devices, child protection and many more, and NHS organisations are expected to implement these. Information can be accessed on the Department of Health website.

The influence of professional and regulatory bodies on standards

The Nursing and Midwifery Council (NMC)

This was established and took over many of the functions of the United Kingdom Central Council for England and Wales. The NMC was set up by the Government to protect the public by ensuring that nurses midwives and health visitors provide high standards of care to their patients. It sets out to achieve this by:

- **Maintaining a register of qualified nurses, midwives and health visitors** to ensure they reach a specific standard on entry to the profession and that professional development and updating to maintain competence continues to enable them to re-register every three years. It also prevents by law anyone calling themselves a nurse who is not registered.
- **Setting standards for education, practice and conduct** necessary for programmes leading to registration and recordable qualifications. The NMC also takes appropriate steps to satisfy itself that the standards have been met.
- **Setting standards and providing guidance to the local supervising authorities for midwives** to ensure women receive high standards of midwifery care.
- **Providing advice for nurses, midwives and health visitors** either by direct enquiries or through a number of useful publications which inform nurses about the standards of their practice, including, advice on developing practice, accepting gifts, confidentiality, records and record keeping, administration of medicines, accountability and many more.
- **Considering allegations of misconduct or unfitness to practice due to ill health** the NMC publishes a code of conduct for nurses, midwives

and health visitors which sets the standards required of all nurses and midwives. The purpose of the code is to:

- inform the professions of the standard of professional conduct required of them in the exercise of their professional accountability
- inform the public, other professions and employers of the standard of professional conduct that they can expect of a registered practitioner.

This forms the basis for considering complaints and allegations of unfitness to practice as a result misconduct or ill health (NMC, 2004). Every nurse is provided with a copy of this.

The Royal College of Nursing

The Royal College of Nursing is a professional body which represents nurses and nursing and aims to promote excellence in practice and shape health policies. For many years it has had a quality improvement programme which has brought together work on clinical guidelines, audit, clinical governance and quality improvement in health care and provided a source of information, guidelines and educational opportunities for its members. Guidelines and best practice have been published in a number of areas including, nurse staffing, continence, manual handling, peri-operative fasting, pain management in children, the management of venous leg ulcers and many more.

Local standards

Local standards can be developed for many areas of practice, for example, mouth care, hygiene, management of acute pain, privacy and dignity and many more. They should incorporate national guidance where this is available.

Reasons for use

Locally developed standards are produced to improve the standard of care to patients. It is helpful if standards are written as this will reduce confusion or misunderstandings about the right or wrong ways of doing things. Written standards:

- help to clarify the scope of nursing functions

- alert the nurse to possible complications, allowing them to prevent adverse patient outcomes
- set parameters of care and demonstrate interdisciplinary needs and expectations of the nursing team
- help to protect the nurse if they are following a practice standard guideline
- outline the importance of patients' and relatives' involvement
- provide a basis for evaluation, teaching, in-service reviews and induction and orientation programmes.

Benefits

There are a number of benefits of developing and implementing standards:

- assists nurses in evaluating and improving their own practice
- provides objective criteria for measuring nurse performance
- contributes to determining staffing needs and skill mix
- identifies research needs
- acts as a good educational tool
- generates a good source of satisfaction when standards are achieved
- improves nursing care and service.

Format

There is no hard and fast rule about the format of standards but the following will provide structure and a standardised approach.

- **Background and statement of intent** This sets the scene for the standard and may include why it is important for the standard to be implemented, the context in which the standard is being used and what the standard is intended to achieve.
- **Assessment criteria** This should include how the patient and their environment are assessed prior to carrying out the interventions of the standard.
- **Intervention** This section provides details of the actions and processes the nurse will take and the ways in which it should be done to ensure the required standard. The interventions should be based on evidence of best practice.
- **Expected outcomes** This should state what should happen as a result of the intervention in the standard.

- **Evaluation and Audit** It is important that the care is evaluated to ensure that patient's outcomes are as expected. The standard should be audited to ensure it is being carried out appropriately (see section below).
- **Glossary of terms** To ensure all readers have a common understanding of what key terms mean.
- **References** So that the evidence base can be checked.
- **Originator, approver and date** To make clear whether the standard is agreed across a department, directorate or the whole organisation and when, so that planned updating can be undertaken.

Audit

An audit tool should be developed with the standard and may include any of the following (specific measurable criteria should be identified):

- review of documentation
- observation of practice
- observation of staff (performance and behaviour)
- review of environment and equipment
- review of medicines' management
- interviews to obtain patients view and/or staff views
- review of management issues.

It may be more objective if the audit is undertaken by a nurse from another area and who has sufficient experience. Action plans should be developed to make improvements.

Role of matron in setting and monitoring standards

The public consultation undertaken to develop the NHS Plan (DoH, 2000) clearly indicated the public's view for the return of the matron figure. They wanted a 'strong clinical leader with clear authority at ward level. Patients and their relatives expressed concern that responsibility for aspects of basic care was too often diffused and that nursing staff were frustrated in their efforts to remedy shortcomings across a range of services and facilities fundamental to patient care' (HSC, 2001). Matrons have a key role in setting, implementing and monitoring standards of professional practice, of clinical care, of cleanliness, hygiene and infection control and of the environment and in assisting and supporting others to achieve these standards. The 10 key things that matrons do are set out in table 16.1. (DoH, Press release 2002)

Table 16.1: 10 key things that matrons do	
1	Lead by example. Matron leads the nursing team in groups of wards demonstrating to other nurses the high standards NHS patients can expect.
2	Make sure patients get quality care. Matrons are responsible for driving up standards of care, ensuring continuous improvement, making sure every patient gets quality care.
3	Make sure wards are clean. Matrons oversee the standards of cleanliness of each of the wards in their charge.
4	Ensure patients' nutritional needs are met. Matrons ensure that patients get their meals and are able to eat them and that the nutritional needs of all patients are met.
5	Prevent and control hospital-acquired infection. Matrons ensure that the highest standards for preventing and controlling infection are set and met on every ward.
6	Improve the wards for patients.
7	Oversee the spending of ward budgets. Each ward sister has a budget of £5,000 to improve the ward environment. Matrons ensure nurses do have their say over how this is spent.
8	Make sure nurses have more power.
9	Empower nurses by enabling them to order tests, admit and discharge patients, triage patients and, where appropriate, prescribe medicines.
10	Make sure patients are treated with respect. Matrons have the power to ensure nurses and other NHS staff treat patients with respect at all times, ensuring privacy and dignity are protected.

Patient and Public Involvement in monitoring standards

Patient and Public Involvement Forums (PPI Forums) are independent statutory bodies established in December 2003 (DoH, 2003). They are made up of local volunteers and representatives of local voluntary organisations and there is a forum for each NHS organisation. Among their responsibilities they are required to:

- monitor and review the range and operation of services provided by NHS trusts
- provide advice, reports and recommendations based on reviews that they carry out
- obtain the views of patients and their carers about the range and operation of services and report those views to the relevant trust.

To carry out these functions the PPI forums are required to visit hospitals and other health care environments. By doing this they are taking on some of the responsibilities previously carried out by the Community Health Councils and they will be involved in public consultation exercises when major changes to health service provision are being planned.

Remember what you can do

- Keep up to date with the national standards produced for your area by looking on the Department of Health as well as professional web sites and reading journals.
- Ensure you are aware of the your requirements in relation to the Professional Code of Conduct.
- Find out what standards are set in your own organisation.
- Find out more about your local Patient and Public Involvement Forum.
- Speak to your matron about the standards for your area.
- Speak to your colleagues and senior nurses if there is a need for a standard in a particular area.
- Offer to participate in the audit and monitoring of standards for your area.

References

DoH (1991) The Patient's Charter. Department of Health, London

DoH (1994) The Maternity Charter. Department of Health, London

DoH (1995) The Patient's Charter and You. Department of Health, London

DoH (1996) Services for children and young people. Department of Health, London

DoH (2000) The NHS Plan. HMSO, London

DoH (2001a) Your Guide to the NHS, Department of Health, London

DoH (2001b) Essence of Care. Patient focused Benchmarking for Health Care Practitioners HMSO, London

DoH (2002) Nearly 2,000 Modern matrons in the NHS – two years early. DoH Press Release 15th April 2002 (Ref 2002/0188)

DoH (2003) Letter to NHS organisations Patient and Public Involvement Forums. Gateway reference 2413 4th December

DoH (2004) Standards for Better Health: Health Care Standards for Services under the NHS – A Consultation. Department of Health, London

Healthcare Commission (2005) Assessment for Improvement. The Annual Healthcheck. Healthcare Commission, London

HSC (1998) National Service Frameworks. 1998/074, 16th April

HSC (2001) Implementing the NHS plan: Modern matrons. Strengthening the role of ward sisters and introducing senior sisters. 2001/010. 4th April

Modernisation Agency (2003) Essence of Care. Patient-focused benchmarks for clinical governance. Department of Health, London

NHS (1990) The NHS and Community Care Act 1990. HMSO, London

NMC (2004) The NMC Code of Professional Conduct. Standards for Conduct Performance and Ethics, London

Additional reading

Castledine G (2001) New benchmarking tool reveals nursing's essence. *Br J Nurs* **10**(6): 410

Chambers N, Jolly A (2002) Essence of Care: Making a difference. *Nurs Standard* **17**(11): 40–4

Dermatology Nursing Standards of Clinical Practice. *Dermatol Nurs* **15**(2):160, 163–4, 167–8

DoH (1999) National Service Framework – Paediatric Intensive Care. DoH, London

DoH (1999) National Service Framework for Mental Health. DoH, London

DoH (2000) National Service Framework for Coronary Heart Disease. DoH, London

DoH (2001) National Service Framework for Older People. DoH. London

DoH (2001) National Service Framework for Diabetes Standards. DoH, London

DoH (2004) National Service Framework for Renal Services Part 1 Dialysis and Transplantation. DoH, London

Useful websites

www.cgsupport.nhs,uk.	Clinical Governance Support Unit
www.dh.gov.uk	Department of Health
www.nice.uk.org	National Institute for Clinical Excellence
www.nmc-uk.org	Nursing and Midwifery Council
www.rcn.org.uk	Royal College of Nursing

Chapter 17

Expanding professional practice

Ann Flavell

The United Kingdom Central Council for Nursing, Midwifery and Health Visiting (UKCC) published its document *The Scope of Professional Practice* (Scope) in 1992. It was intended as a developmental means for nurses to expand the boundaries of practice and promote holistic nursing care. The guidance in this document has been incorporated into the NMC Code of Professional conduct in Standards for Conduct Performance and Ethics (NMC 2004). This chapter describes how roles can be extended and expanded and the safeguards that must be put in place to protect the patient's safety, the standard of nursing care and the nurse in developing their role.

Extended role

Prior to Scope, nurses 'extended' their role by undertaking some tasks previously preformed by doctors. The extended role of the nurse is one 'where tasks are borrowed from other professions, used at the discretion and convenience of others and involves training, supervision and certification by other professions' (Mitchinson and Goodlad, 1996).

The extent to which nurses could make their own decisions about which additional tasks they could perform, or had to do, varied from hospital to hospital. This meant that nurses could only use skills for which they had local approval, regardless of their competence and previous experience.

Role expansion

Role expansion refers to nurses carrying out activities not included in their normal training for registration. Therefore nurses must be aware of the boundaries of their own knowledge and skills and only undertake care for which they are prepared, competent and confident.

> *If an aspect of practice is beyond your level of competence or outside your area of registration, you must obtain help and supervision from a competent practitioner until you and your employer consider that you have acquired the requisite knowledge and skills.*

(NMC, 2004)

Purpose of the expansion of practice

- Expanding practice provides nurses with the opportunity to be innovative resulting in confident practice and extended role. Consequently, more flexible and efficient care to patients is intended.
- The framework aims to guide nurses to decide what roles they can expand and develop. It provides the opportunity to cross all professional boundaries to enhance patient care resulting in a more forward thinking establishment with better team working between all disciplines.
- Some nurses have viewed role expansion as undertaking previous doctors' roles but its intention is to improve patient care in all aspects. It can be used to guide nurses in new and unique developments.
- It provides the opportunity to progress the nursing profession as a whole and not simply to alleviate doctors of their more menial tasks.

The key principles must always be explored to ensure patient care is best provided.

Key principles

The Code of Professional Conduct recognises that every nurse, midwife and specialist community public health nurse is accountable for their practice and that it is their professional judgement that can provide innovative solutions to meeting the needs of patients/clients in a health service that is constantly changing.

The six principles that underpin taking on responsibility beyond the traditional boundaries of practice are that the nurse/midwife must:

- be satisfied that each aspect of practice is directed to meeting the needs and serving the interests of the patient/client
- endeavour always to achieve, maintain and develop knowledge, skill and competence to respond to those needs and interests
- honestly acknowledge any limits of personal knowledge and skill and take steps to remedy any relevant deficits in order to meet the needs of patients/clients effectively and appropriately
- ensure that existing nursing care is not compromised by new developments and responsibilities
- acknowledge personal accountability
- avoid any inappropriate delegation.

By addressing these key principles nurses have a powerful tool to support their argument to develop and improve patient services. Whatever the development is, the necessary skills within those roles must be recognised and co-ordinated to offer a consistent standard in expanding roles. Professional experience, enthusiasm and intuition, as well as education and supervision are important.

To ensure nurses are prepared, competent and confident, there need to be systems in place which provide clear guidelines, support and appropriate training for nurses to effectively expand roles.

Implementation of expanded roles

If a new role is to be developed or an existing role to be expanded, then the nurse/nurses in that role should be supported to do so by the organisation in which they work within a defined area of clinical practice. It may or may not be appropriate for the role to be transferred into other areas.

Prior to any new role a process of discussion should be entered into with the senior nurses and colleagues in the multidisciplinary team and agreement reached for the development of practice.

The key principles should be accounted for by meeting the following criteria:

- The role should enhance improve patient/client care.
- The role must be appropriate for that area.
- The nurse must be able to demonstrate an understanding of the new role to the satisfaction of their ward/department manager or senior nurse.
- The knowledge and skill base required for the role must be defined and achieved.
- There must be a willingness to undertake the role.

- The individual must be appropriately trained and assessed as competent in practice and have the underpinning knowledge.

Therefore a framework for the development of any roles for nurses should be clear and supported by the organisation they work for.

Framework for the development of a new role

The framework ensures that all those undertaking role expansion have the appropriate level of knowledge, judgement and skills to allow them to practice effectively and safely.

Each framework should comprise of:

A definition of the activity

This gives details of the new role, the circumstances and conditions under which the nurse can undertake the role and the details of the level of training required.

An outline of the procedure

This provides the practitioner with the information on the technique based on best evidence-based practice. This practical procedure information can be used as a measure for benchmarking best practice standard.

How competence is assessed.

Details of self- and peer-assessment relating to the quality and quantity of learning knowledge and skills of the particular activity will be evident in this section. The peer assessor will be a clinical expert willing to provide supervision and assessment and who has previously undergone the training agreed and is considered actively proficient in the activity.

Self-assessment is used to encourage self-reflection and role development to build from novice to expert. Accountability lies with the practitioner to ensure they are competent and confident to undertake the new role.

The frequency of assessment and supervision of scope of practice should be negotiated between the individual clinical expert, who has previously undergone the training agreed and is considered proficient in the activity and the department manager.

Impact of expanding roles on nursing practice

There has been much written as to the value of expanding roles in practice.

Disadvantages

- Following the reduction of junior doctors' hours, Castledine (1993) and Denner (1995) queried whether nurses were becoming doctors' handmaids.
- Marsden (1995) feared that some nurses could ingratiate themselves with their medical colleagues whom they perceive as superior.
- Role expansion has been perceived by some as an increased burden on already hard-pressed staff and that the basic and fundamental aspects of nursing are compromised as a result. Tasks previously done by doctors are not necessarily more important. Equally they do not necessarily require more knowledge and skills than nursing activities.

Advantages

- It can be a way of helping nurses to develop necessary skills, knowledge, become more analytical, critical and flexible and be proactive rather than reactive to patients' needs.
- It can help to clarify specialist roles and increase nurse satisfaction.
- Competence assessment can assist in advancing through a clinical career structure.
- Patients receive high quality care more quickly in some circumstances.

With these views in mind, it is vital to ensure that the benefits of new role developments will outweigh the disadvantages and that the nurse undertaking expansion is valued and recognised for the improved service provision. While the individual is accountable and responsible for their actions, an agreed framework is essential.

Conclusion

With the rapid changes in healthcare and increased intensity and complexity of care nurses will continue to expand their knowledge and skills. To maintain safe practices they must be prepared, competent and confident in their challenging roles and only those who have the required knowledge skills and aptitude to undertake expanded roles should perform these tasks.

Trusts must provide resources and bear responsibility for expansion of skills. The support and guidance for staff through the change development process should be available. Education and training that clearly identifies the knowledge and skills required should be available to ensure the practice is research based, current and reliable. Additionally, the way competence and supervision is assessed needs to be clear to ensure safe practice.

The assumption that all those who are trained in the knowledge and skills of a new practice does not provide either the individual or the organisation in which they work with the confidence that their practice is safe. It is therefore essential to make sure that any new skill is supervised and assessed by a competent person who will determine whether or not their practice is safe.

Each individual nurse is responsible for their own actions or omissions and the organisations they work for have a responsibility to accept vicarious liability so long as the nurse acts to the required standard. Therefore it is vital that the nurse is fully aware of the framework for any new role and ensures that the knowledge and skills learnt are maintained in the clinical setting.

New roles give the nursing profession the opportunity to expand and develop. It can open gates in all areas of patient care for the individual nurse to be creative, innovative and to build on personal strengths and weaknesses.

Developing practice in this way should be judged upon its ability to contribute to improving standards of patient care and this rightly should be how it is considered.

Remember what you can do

- Read your local policy on expanding practice and remember the six principles that underpin expansion of practice.
- Find out what expanding roles can be done in your area and what preparation you need to do to undertake the roles and safeguard patient care.
- Discuss with your colleagues if there are any other areas for role expansion in your specialty that will enhance patient care.

References

NMC (2004) Code of Professional Conduct: Standards for Conduct, Performance and Ethics. Nursing and Midwifery Council, London

Castledine G (1993) Has the Scope of professional practice failed in its original aim? *Br J Nurs* **4**(21): 1279

Denner S (1995) Extending professional practice: benefits and pitfalls. *Nurs Times* **91**(14): 27–9

Marsden J (1995) Setting up nurse practitioner roles: issues in practice. *Br J Nurs* **4**(16): 948–53

Mitchinson S, Goodlad S (1996) Changes in the roles and responsibilities of nurses. *Prof Nurs* **11**(11) 734–6

United Kingdom Central Council for Nursing, Midwifery and Health Visiting (UKCC) 1992a The Scope of Professional Practice. UKCC, London

Additional reading

Edwards J (2000) Intra-articular or soft tissue injections by nurses: preparation for expanded practice. *Nurs Standard* **14**(33): 43–6

Edward K (1995) What are nurses views on expanding practice. *Nurs Standard* **9**(41): 38–40

Higgins M (1997) Developing and supporting expansion of the nurse's role. *Nurs Standard* **11**(24): 41–4

Jones A (2003) Changes in practice at the nurse-doctor interface. Using focus groups to explore the perceptions of first level nurses working in acute care settings. *J Clin Nurs* **12**(1): 124–31

Leonard S (1999) The expanded role of the registered nurse: Studying nurses perceptions. *Nurs Standard* **13**(43): 32–6

Marsden J (2000) A real eye opener. *Nurs Standard* **14**(42): 61

UKCC (2000) Perception of the Scope of Professional Practice. 1st January UKCC, London

UKCC (2000) Enrolled Nursing, Delivering the Agenda for Action. 1st January UKCC, London

Useful websites

www.nmc-uk.org   Nursing and Midwifery Council
www.modern.nhs.uk   Modernisation Agency
www.dh.gov.uk   Department of Health

Chapter 18

Research and evidence-based nursing

Rebecca Jester

This chapter aims to demystify research related to clinical care and to provide a basic introduction on how to use research and evidence to underpin your practice. Also it provides an overview of the systems available to support nurses conducting clinically-based research projects. This chapter does not provide an in-depth research text, but rather a practical introduction to some of the main issues of relevance to nurses which includes:

- Defining research and evidence-based practice.
- How to critically evaluate research and implement it into practice.
- How to get help when planning and conducting research projects.
- The importance of publishing research findings and tips on getting published.

Background

Despite the fact that evidence-based nursing did not gain widespread adoption until the 1990s, nurses have been using research to underpin their practice since the 19th century.

> *In dwelling upon the vital importance of sound observation, it must never be lost sight of what observation is for. It is not for the sake of piling up miscellaneous information or curious facts, but for the sake of saving life and increasing health and comfort.*

(Florence Nightingale, 1859)

During the Crimean war Florence Nightingale collected data on morbidity and mortality rates of wounded soldiers and analysed the data to ascertain if there was a relationship between delay in operating and post-surgical survival.

The genesis of evidence-based nursing practice is in part a response to the need to provide cost effective, high quality care (DoH, 1996). Ritualistic practice is no longer acceptable. While not all nurses are prepared academically to undertake research, all nurses must have an awareness and appreciation of research and how to implement appropriate findings in their everyday practice. As a staff nurse working in the hospital setting, it is important to have an understanding of what research and evidence-based practice are and how to implement them into practice.

Defining research and evidence-based practice

Research may be defined as a systematic process of data collection for the purpose of prediction or explanation and to increase the body of knowledge in a particular area of practice. Practitioners sometimes find it difficult to differentiate between research and audit in clinical practice. The important difference is that research is an attempt to identify new facts and the relationship between them, rather than a simple monitoring of what is happening and comparing it to agreed standards. Both research and audit have their place in contemporary health care. Like nursing care research is a process. The research process comprises a number of key stages as detailed below:

Stage 1   The idea - often borne out of a clinical problem.
Stage 2   Formulation of a research question or hypothesis.
Stage 3   Review of the literature – is there sufficient robust research already to address the idea or solve the problem? If the answer is no this provides the justification for your project.
Stage 4   Refining the research question or hypothesis to reflect new knowledge from the review of literature.
Stage 5   Decide on the most appropriate research method, eg experimental trial, action research, qualitative methods such as phenomenology or grounded theory etc.
Stage 6   Formulating a research proposal, seeking ethical approval from the organisation's ethics committee and registering the project with the research and development department if appropriate.
Stage 7   Collection of data once ethical approval has been gained, eg distributing questionnaires or conducting interviews or focus groups. Ethical principles of confidentiality and consent must be adhered to as agreed with the Ethics Committee and under the conditions of research governance.
Stage 8   Analysis of the data collected using either descriptive and/or inferential statistics or qualitative methods such as thematic or content analysis.

Stage 9   Writing up findings and disseminating via internal reports and external publication at conferences or within professional journals.

In reality it is not always possible to underpin all of your practice with robust research findings. This is because there are gaps in the research-based literature and often it takes many years for findings from substantial clinical trials to be published. Also you may find conflicting research findings on the same subject as the research base on a clinical topic may be inconclusive. Therefore you sometimes need to look for other sources of information and evidence to underpin your practice and policies. Evidence based nursing is described by Sackett et al (1996) as nursing decisions based on:

- best available evidence
- value of clinical experience
- patients' preference.

This suggests there are a number of sources of evidence nurses can use to underpin their practice. A summary of types of evidence can be found in the box below:

Types of evidence

❖ Evidence from research – carrying out a search of published and unpublished literature and using systematic reviews. Including guidelines and protocols developed using empirical evidence.
❖ Evidence based on experiences – reflecting on practice and using non-research publications such as case studies to facilitate discussion on best practice.
❖ Evidence based on theory that is not research based – formal education, symposia and conference presentations.
❖ Evidence gathered from clients and/or their carers about issues of satisfaction/dissatisfaction/complaint and audit data about untoward incidents.

Adapted from le May (1999)

In recent years a number of organisations have developed resources to assist practitioners in developing evidence-based practice via systematic reviews, databases and best practice guidelines. Examples include:

- The Cochrane Library, incorporating the Cochrane database of systematic reviews, the Cochrane controlled trials register and the Cochrane review methodology database.

- The Midwifery Information and Resource Service (MIDIRS).
- NHS Centre for reviews and dissemination and literature searching facilities such as Medline, Psyclit
- The Cumulative Index of Nursing and Allied Health Literature (CINAHL).

One of the most useful tips to give you in this chapter is make full use of the services of your organisation's library services. Librarians will assist you in requesting inter-library loans and help you to conduct literature searches.

How to critically evaluate research and implement it into practice

It must not be assumed that all research, guidelines and publications in professional journals are valid and reliable. Nurses must be able to critically review evidence to assess its validity before basing their practice upon it. A summary of the questions to ask about research papers to ascertain their validity can be found below:

General questions to ask about research papers

- ❖ Was the study clear?
- ❖ Was the research question or hypothesis clearly stated?
- ❖ Was the rationale for the study identified?
- ❖ Did the research design and methods fit the purpose?
- ❖ Was the literature review relevant and systematic?
- ❖ Were the threats to reliability and validity acknowledged and controlled?
- ❖ Were methods of analysis clear and appropriate?
- ❖ Do the findings address the research question or hypothesis?
- ❖ Are the implications for practice acknowledged?
- ❖ Do the conclusions fit with data presented?
- ❖ Are ethical considerations discussed?
- ❖ Who undertook the research?
- ❖ Who funded the work?
- ❖ Do you have enough information to repeat the study?

(Adapted from DePoy and Gitlin, 1994)

DiCenso et al (1998) suggest that:

> ...*in practising evidence based nursing, a nurse has to decide whether the evidence is relevant for the particular patient. The incorporation of clinical expertise should be balanced with the risks and benefits of alternative treatment for each patient and should take into account the patient's unique clinical circumstances, including co-morbid conditions and preferences*

(p 38)

An example of application of the above quotation is the use of full-length anti-embolic stockingd in preventing deep vein thrombosis following lower limb surgery eg total hip replacement. However, in taking into account the patient's individual needs, you may discover that either the patient has a co-morbid state that prohibits the use of anti-embolic stockings or finds them so uncomfortable that they roll them down, increasing the risk of vascular complications. This example demonstrates the necessity for nurses to view evidence-based practice in the context of individual holistic nursing care.

How to get help when planning and conducting research projects

It is important to remember you are not alone in your quest to implement evidence-based practice and seeking support and guidance is essential. To overcome potential barriers and to maximise success in the implementation of evidence-based practice there are many opportunities for support including:

- Finding out if your organisation has a research and development department. If so they can offer you support and guidance in developing research proposals and conducting your project.
- Your local ethics committee will provide you with feedback on your proposed research to ensure it is robust and ethically acceptable.
- In addition, you may get specific support for nurses from the director of nursing and other senior nurses and research nurses
- Ensure you familiarise yourself with the organisation's research governance policy. It provides essential information on your responsibilities when proposing and conducting research.
- Seek support and collaboration from clinical colleagues who have prior experience and expertise in conducting research. For example, clinical nurse specialists, lecturer practitioners and medical colleagues.

- Support for funding projects can be found from professional organisations such as the Royal College of Nursing, Theatre Nurses' Association and Department of Health (details are on websites).

Implementing evidence-based practice involves management of change. Remember to keep people informed of what you are trying to do, seek collaboration and guidance. You may encounter barriers to implementing evidence- based practice including:

- **Negative staff attitudes**: lack of motivation, resistance to change, fear and ritualised practice.
- **Organisation issues**: time, resources, pressure of work and too much change.
- **Educational issues**: unable to access research, lack of knowledge and skill in research appraisal, language of research makes it inaccessible .
- **Cooperation issues:** medical colleagues may block implementation, other professions believing nursing research is sub-standard

However, by seeking appropriate support and guidance as detailed earlier, these barriers can be overcome. Good communication and collaboration is the key!

Publishing research findings

The thought of presenting your research findings at a conference or in a professional journal may appear daunting, but you have an ethical obligation to share good practice and disseminate your findings not just locally, but to practitioners in other organisations. Also you will get a real sense of professional self-worth when you see you name in print.

Some frequently asked questions and answers about getting published are presented below.

What sort of things can I publish?

- original research.
- literature reviews
- opinion pieces
- book reviews
- conference abstracts.

How should I structure a research paper?

- the title should convey succinctly and accurately what your paper is about
- identification of key words: these are used for key word searches
- authors' details and main contact
- abstract or summary: 100–200 words – brief overview of aim, procedure, results and implications.

Main paper

- introduction: background and context of the paper
- literature review
- theoretical explanation from the literature review
- rationale for your own research.

Method

- design: eg random controlled trials, quasi-experimental, survey, phenomenological. Give the rationale for the method chosen and rejection of other approaches.

Subjects

- include the size of the sample, the type of sampling method and data regarding the subjects eg. age, gender, ethnicity etc.

Apparatus/materials

- the tools used: questionnaires, index, measuring apparatus etc. and how validity, reliability was established.

Procedure

- it is best to summarise in a table or time-line – who did what, to whom and where.

Results

- use graphs, tables and charts that are clearly labelled. You must state what statistical tests were used and what the actual values were. What your 'p' value was taken as. Usually figures are presented on a separate page at the end of the manuscript and you indicate in the text where you want the figures placed.

Discussion

- start with the re-statement of your findings and then go on to relate to how your findings affirm or refute previous findings
- you must produce a feasible theoretical explanation for your findings and implications for practice or policy
- include ethical considerations, limitations and acknowledgements
- referencing you can use Harvard system, but check contributor guidelines. They are very particular about how references are presented and may reject you if an incorrect format is used. Also when ever possible use up-to-date reference material.

See below for some useful tips on maximising your success in getting published.

General tips on getting your work published

❖ Think carefully about which journal to write for.
❖ Only submit to one journal at a time.
❖ Remember that your first draft will certainly not be the final manuscript.
❖ Follow the journal's notes to contributors very carefully for structure, style and level of content.
❖ Think carefully about co-authors and acknowledgement of contributors.
❖ Review several recent copies of the journal you are writing for to get a feel for the level (impact value) and type of paper they publish.
❖ Remember conference presentations that have been subjected to peer review count as publications.
❖ Remember to get prior permission for reproduction of any photos or figures etc.
❖ Remember it can take anything up to 2 years to see your paper in print.
❖ Expect rejection and use it as a learning exercise.
❖ Don't give up if rejected, take on board the referees' comments and re-vamp and submit to another journal.
❖ First attempt – wise to co-publish with an experienced author.

Conclusion

This chapter has attempted to provide an introductory guide to the understanding and use of research and evidence to underpin practice. A number of potential barriers to evidence-based practice have been highlighted and practical tips on how to implement research into practice have been provided. The most important message from this chapter is that you are not alone in trying to promote evidence based practice. There are many sources of support available to you in most organisations including:

- a robust research governance policy
- a well established research and development department
- specific support for nurses in developing research ideas and formulating proposals for ethical approval
- well resourced library facilities
- informal support from experienced researchers.

Remember what you can do

- Find out the sources of evidence you can use to underpin your practice.
- Use the resources available to help you develop evidence.
- Ask your librarian for help.
- Ask senior nursing and other clinical colleagues for help.
- Learn how to critically review evidence and assess its validity before basing practice on it.
- Find out what support is available to you in your own organisation.

References

Department of Health (1996) Promoting Clinical Effectiveness: A Framework for Action in and Through the NHS. NHSE, Leeds

DePoy E, Gitlin L (1994) Introduction to Research. Multiple Strategies for Health and Human Services. Mosby, St Louis

DiCenso A, Cullum N, Ciliska D (1998) Implementing evidence-based nursing: some misconceptions. *Evidence-based Nurs* **1**(2): 38–40

Le May A (1999) Evidence–based practice. Nursing Times Monographs No 1. Nursing Times Books, London

Nightingale F (1859) Notes on Nursing. Lippincott, Philadelphia

Sackett D, Rosenberg W, Muir Gray J (1996) Evidence-based medicine: what it is and what it isn't. *Br Med J* **312**(7023): 71–2

Additional reading

Dempsey PA, Dempsey AD (2000) Using Nursing Research: Process, Critical Evaluation and Utilization. Lippincott, Philadelphia

Hek G, Judd M, Moule P (2002) Making Sense of Research: An Introduction for Health and Social Care Practitioners. Continuum, London

Polit DF, Tatano Beck C, Hungler BP (2001) Essentials of Nursing Research: Methods, Appraisal, and Utilization. Lippincott, Philadelphia

Useful websites

www.dh.gov.uk   National Electronic Library for Health
www.internurse.com   Online archive of peer-reviewed articles
www.natn.org.uk   National Association of Theatre Nurses
www.nelh.nhs.uk   National Electronic Library for Health
www.rcn.org.uk   Royal college of Nursing

Chapter 19
Clinical information

Ann Close

Information is an essential part of health care today and for delivery of the NHS Modernisation agenda. It is used in:

- the organisation, management and delivery of healthcare
- the employment and management of staff
- performance management including monitoring of financial, activity and quality targets.

Information strategy

As part of its plan for modernisation of the NHS, the Government developed an information strategy to be implemented between 1998 and 2005 to ensure information is used to help patients receive the best possible care (NHS Executive, 1998). This strategy should help you use and manage information more effectively.

The aims of the strategy are:

- To ensure that patients can be confident that professionals have reliable and rapid access to information.
- To eliminate any unnecessary travel or delay to treatment by providing remote on-line access to services.
- To provide patients with access to information and advice about their condition, about lifestyles and the health service.
- To provide NHS professionals with on-line access to national evidence and guidance about treatment.
- To ensure availability of accurate information for managers to monitor performance.

Using this strategy as a blueprint, most NHS organisations have developed a local information strategy which provides a vision and direction of how information and information technology will be developed to support patient care and the delivery of services in the future within the organisation or health economy. You should try and read this to understand what your local plans are and how it will impact on the delivery of care in your area.

Information for nurses

Information is vital in helping you to deal with the complexities of your working life. It is used for:

- assessing, planning, delivering and monitoring patient care
- ensuring high standards of care and developing policies and evidence-based practice
- personal and professional development
- auditing and monitoring practice
- managing and organising ward and department activities
- research purposes.

It is necessary to help you make decisions about what you should do and how you can work effectively.

Assessing, planning, delivering and monitoring patient care

Information is gathered from patients, and sometimes family and friends, through discussions and observation or is provided through correspondence and records from other health care professionals. This information is used by nurses to:

- identify problems and priorities for care
- identify things that are important to or of concern to the patient and their family
- identify goals and plan care.

Subsequently information is used in:

- documenting what has been carried out, progress made and the outcomes of the care given
- making decisions about future care such as whether to refer the patient to therapy or how to treat a pressure sore.

When collecting the information it is important to:

- co-ordinate what information is available so that the patient is only asked for the same information once
- only ask for information that is relevant
- ensure that existing information is used, ie from the patients' records from other members of the healthcare team
- use appropriate ways of communicating with patients depending on the setting and the situation.

High standards of care and developing evidence-based practice

Information is essential to help develop policies, procedures, guidelines and standards of care which will guide staff in their work. Up-to-date best practice can be obtained through information on the internet, or issued through bodies such as NICE (National Institute for Clinical Excellence) from professional bodies such as, the Nursing and Midwifery Council, the Royal Colleges and from journals. Evidence from local and national audits will also provide useful information to influence these practices.

Research purposes

The value of research in underpinning clinical practice is stressed by NICE but bridging the gap between research and practice is not always easy. Nurses need to know where they can find out about relevant research and they need to know how to make sense of the evidence they find. This requires an understanding of research processes including data collection and analysis methods and the ability to evaluate research findings, otherwise it will be impossible to make an informed judgement about its relevance and rigour.

Auditing and monitoring practice

Information is collected and analysed through a range of audits such as:

- infection control audits, which many look at hand washing, disposal of sharps, handling of linen, general cleanliness and many more
- patient surveys to determine what they feel about aspects of their stay in hospital, their care and treatmen
- audit of aspects of care such as charting and record keeping, pressure sores, wound healing and more
- health and safety audits.

Information from audits is analysed to indicate the level of performance achieved and gives the opportunity to plan actions to make more improvements.

Managing and organising ward and department activities

Information is required:

- To manage staff to deliver care including:
  - rostering and deployment
  - employment, including contracts, personal records, training records
  - performance management, appraisal, sickness and absence monitoring.
- To ensure there are sufficient resources:
  - stores and stocks
  - maintenance of equipment
  - catering
  - linen supplies.
- For staff and patients:
  - ward or department profiles which describe the ward and what it offers
  - visiting times.

Personal and professional development

The Code of Professional Conduct (NMC, 2004) requires all registered nurses and midwives to maintain their professional knowledge and competence throughout their working lives. This is to ensure:

- they deliver lawful, safe and effective practice without direct supervision
- they deliver care based on current evidence, best practice and, where applicable, research
- they can facilitate students and others to develop their confidence.

This requires continuous personal and professional development. Information from many sources is required to support this.

Communicating information

This is mostly done by verbal communication, or from records and documentation and occurs at all levels in formal and informal situations, for example in discussion with patients and staff, telephone calls with colleagues and relatives, through ward meetings and handover reports and from patients' records and care plans.
It is therefore important that information communicated is:

- accurate, clear and concise so that others can understand, it should be free of jargon and abbreviations unless it is clear everyone is familiar with those used
- relevant to the purpose and timely
- accessible to others
- recorded systematically so that it can be easily located by others
- easily transferred with the patient
- is kept confidential.

Documenting and recording information

In nursing, documenting and recording information is an essential and integral part of the care process but it is sometimes seen as less important than hands-on delivery. The United Kingdom Central Council (UKCC) highlighted its concern and indicated that:

> ... There is substantial evidence to indicate that inadequate and inappropriate record keeping concerning the care of patients and clients neglects their interests

(UKCC 1993)

The council published its *Standards for Records and Record Keeping* in a document which sets out every registered nurse's accountability and responsibility. This has been reviewed and revised by the NMC and published as Guidelines for Records and Record keeping (2005)

Many organisations have local policies for recording and documenting information about patients and their care. You should check these out for your own area of work.

Information technology

Traditionally, clinical information has been recorded in the patient's health record. This may be in the medical notes or nursing documentation or a combined record. However, increasingly information is being recorded in an electronic format.

The Electronic Health Record is a record of life-long, core clinical information with eventual electronic transfer of patient records between GPs.

The Electronic Patient Record is a record of information about the care a patient has received in an organisation and is held on computer systems instead of paper. This enables professionals to access and add to the record.

The aim is that records can then be integrated across health and social care settings and follow patients rather than be organisation specific.

Initially the 1998 strategy required all acute hospitals to have EPR in place by April 2005 but a new strategy (DoH, 2002) pushed back the existing targets and trusts must now have 'elements' of systems in place by 2005.

Access to health records

Patients now have the legal right to access their health records. The Data Protection Act 1984 gave them the right to access their computer held records and the Access to Health Record Act 1990 gave them the right to access their manual records. More recent legislation, the Data Protection Act, 1998, covers paper based information too.

In addition to patients having access, the records may be inspected in the event of an internal complaint or used as evidence in a court of law. Nurses therefore who contribute to patients' records must be aware of this and give careful consideration to the language, terminology and content they use. Information recorded should be used to enhance patient care and be honest and objective.

Confidentiality of information

The Nursing and Midwifery Council's Code of Professional Conduct(NMC, 2004) outlines the expectations of a registered nurse and midwife in keeping information confidential.
In section five it states:

As a registered nurse or midwife you must protect confidential information

5.1

You must treat information about patients and clients as confidential and use it only for the purposes for which it was given..........
You must guard against breaches of confidentiality by protecting information from improper disclosure at all times.

5.2

You should seek patients' and clients' wishes regarding sharing of information with their family and others. When a patient or client is considered incapable of giving permission, you should consult relevant colleagues.

5.3

If you are required to disclose information outside the team, that will have personal consequences for patients or clients, you must obtain their consent. If the patient or client withholds consent or if consent cannot be obtained disclosure may be made only where:
* *They can be justified in the public interest*
* *They are required by law or by order of a court*

5.4

Where there is an issue of child protection you must act at all times in accordance with national and local policies

The Department of Health issued guidance on *The Protection and Use of Patient Information* in March 1996. (DoH, 1996). This sets out the basic principles of keeping patients informed and safeguarding information. The Chief Medical Officer of England commissioned a review of all patient-identifiable information which passes from the NHS in England to other NHS or non NHS bodies and this became know as the Caldicott Report (1997). Subsequently each NHS organisation has had to appoint a senior health professional to act as Caldicott

Guardian to oversee the processes for agreeing, monitoring and reviewing protocols governing access to patient-identifiable information by staff.

Security of information

Security of information is of prime importance and there are simple steps that can be taken.

For electronically held records:

- using individual passwords which should not be shared with others
- giving levels of access to computer-held information dependent on the work of the individual
- frequent changing of passwords
- closing down when leaving the computer.

For paper based records:

- keeping records in designated places either in locked cupboards, rooms or under the constant scrutiny of a member of staff
- having safe systems for the transfer of notes to other locations
- checking with visiting staff to the ward that they have the authority to see any records
- keeping patients care plans in places which are accessible to patients and staff but not to their visitors or other patients
- ensuring informal notes and jottings are destroyed or stored securely.

For verbal communication:

- ensure telephone conversations are held in privacy
- where possible have discussions with patients in private areas
- ensure handover reports keep information confidential.

Patients' access to information

Patients are provided with more information that ever before. Recent government policy has recognised the importance of patients having more information about the services available to them and how the health service and its healthcare professionals are performing. Patients themselves have also demanded that they have information about what is happening to them and what they can expect from healthcare professionals. Professionals, too, recognise that patients need more information to enable them to make decisions, give informed consent and participate in and take responsibility for their own care.

Accessing information is much easier now through:

• the internet
• information materials provided by hospitals and GPs
• information provided by patient, voluntary and charity groups
• government published materials
• TV, newspapers and magazines.

As a result there is more demand for qualified nurses to keep up to date with new information and not rely on information acquired several years ago. You can do this by using many of the databases that are accessible through the internet. (See useful databases below)

Help is also usually at hand through your local library facilities.

Remember what you can do

■ Ask your line manager about the organisation's or directorate's information strategy or plan.
■ Discuss with your colleagues the information needed to organise your ward/department and manage patient care effectively. Do you have all the information you need? Do you collect information that you don't use?
■ Consider if there is anything you can do to manage the information you need more effectively.
■ Do you need to take any action to improve communication, documentation or record keeping?
■ Make sure you are aware of your organisation's plans for electronic records.
■ Make sure you know what to do if a patient asks for access to their health records.

- Discuss with your colleagues if the measurers taken to ensure confidentiality and security of information are adequate. What else could be done?
- Make sure you are up to date with the NMC Code of Professional Conduct.
- Make sure you know how to access information from your library, the internet and your local intranet.

References

Department of Health (2002) Delivering 21st Century IT support for the NHS: Integrated Care Records Service. London DoH

Department of Health (1996) Health Service Guideline: The Protection and Use of Patient Information HSG (96) 18/LASSL (96) 5 March 1996

NHS Executive (1998) Information for Health – An Information Strategy for the Modern NHS 1998-2005. NHS Executive: London

Nursing and Midwifery Council (2004) Code of Professional Conduct. NMC, London

Nursing and Midwifery Council (2005) Guidelines for Records and Record Keeping. NMC, London

The Access to Health Records Act (1990)

The Caldicott Committee (1997) Report on the Review of Patient-Identifiable Information, Department of Health, London

The Data Protection Act 1984

The Data Protection Act 1998

United Kingdom Central Council for Nursing Midwifery and Health Visiting (1993) Standards for Records and Record Keeping

Additional reading

Washer P (2002) Professional networking using computer-mediated communication. *Br J Nurs* **11**(18): 1215–18

Useful websites

www.dh.gov.uk   Department of Health
http://biomed.niss.ac.uk   Wish Database Site

www.nice.org.uk	National Institute for Clinical Excellence
www.midirs.org	Midwives Information and Resource Service
www.nelh.nhs.uk	National Electronic Library for Health
www.nmc-uk.org	Nursing and Midwifery Council
www.rcn.org.uk	Royal College of Nursing
www.audit-commission.gov.uk	Audit Commission
www.nao.gov.uk	National Audit Office
www.npfit.nhs.uk	National Programme for IT
www.ic.nhs.uk	Health and Social Centre Information Centre

Section 4
Professional issues

You as a nurse in a hospital

The patients' and public's expectations for improvements in the quality of services delivered in hospitals was highlighted in the last section. Just as their expectations of care are greater nowadays so are their expectations of you as a nurse and the colleagues you work with. Not only do they expect high quality care but they expect it to be delivered by knowledgeable, skilled professionals who are also kind, courteous, friendly and polite and who will ensure their privacy and who will respect them.

In addition to raised patient and public expectations there are increased demands from the profession and from NHS organisations. They require more flexibility so that nurses can work in different situations to meet the ever changing needs of patients and to fill shortfalls in skills and availability of staff from other professions. In addition nurses are required to undertake much more than patient care in their own ward. You are probably expected to assess and manage risks, prepare reports, undertake research, teach a range of other staff and students, prepare information materials, manage resources, ensure equipment is maintained, survey patients and colleagues and much more. It is no longer acceptable to complete pre-registration training and do no more. Instead it is essential to gain and update further knowledge and skills to help you become expert practitioners, managers and leaders in the clinical setting.

The expectations of the public, employers and professional bodies extend beyond the workplace. A certain standard of behaviour and conduct is required of you outside the hospital and within your private life. Nurses are seen by many members of the public to have a certain standing in the community and their confidence in the profession is diminished if these standards of behaviour are flouted. The Nursing and Midwifery Council gives clear guidance on its requirements with this regard in the Code of Professional Conduct (NMC 2002)

This section aims to help you think about what your role and responsibilities are and what others expect from you both inside and outside hospitals and work settings. It also looks at how you can develop the knowledge, skills and behaviours required and get support in doing this.

Chapter 20 Legal issues. This will help you understand accountability. In addition it examines the legal aspects of registration and what vicarious liability means in reality. It also covers some legal aspects of care that are of concern to nurses in hospitals including medicines management and consent to treatment.

Chapter 21 Professional Nursing and Midwifery Practice examines the role of the Nursing and Midwifery Council and the Code of Professional Conduct and also interprets the functions of registration and regulation. *Chapter 22 Clinical support.* This chapter provides an overview of the types of support available in clinical settings which will help you improve knowledge and skills and maintain and develop practice. It includes preceptorship, mentoring clinical supervision, practice based education and stress management. *Chapter 23 Continuing professional development (CPD)* examines the benefits of CPD and looks at how you can take responsibility for developing a portfolio, contributing effectively to appraisals and taking up opportunities offered. *Chapter 24 Career Development* builds on the previous chapter and looks at how to plan and develop your career and use opportunities available. It examines the key skills to success, how to get started and where to get help and support.

References

NMC (2002) Code of Professional Conduct. NMC, London

Chapter 20
Legal issues

Bridgit Dimond

Of necessity this chapter is an extremely concise summary of some of the principles of law which apply to the staff nurse and it is recommended that readers should refer to the author's textbook for more detail and for other topics on relevant law (Dimond, 2004).

Accountability

If a practitioner has caused harm to a patient, she might be held accountable in four different courts/tribunals or hearings: criminal, civil, disciplinary proceedings and fitness to practice proceedings.

Criminal

Any health professional who has acted with such gross negligence as to cause the death of a patient could be found guilty of manslaughter. The hearing would take place in the crown court (following committal proceedings held in the magistrates court) and if the practitioner pleaded not guilty, the case would be heard before a jury who, in order to convict the defendant of manslaughter would have to find the facts of gross negligence and causation (ie the negligence caused the death) proved by the evidence beyond reasonable doubt. The leading case is that of R. v Adomako where an anaesthetist was held guilty of manslaughter following the death of a patient on an operating theatre table.

Criminal proceedings could also be possible as a result of offences under Health and Safety legislation. Section 7 of the Health and Safety Act 1974 which requires employees to take reasonable care for the health and safety of himself and of others who may be affected by his acts or omissions at work and also to co-operate with the employer in implementing health and safety duties.

A practitioner may also be required to give evidence in criminal cases involving colleagues as the colleagues of Dr Shipman had to do.

Civil liability

Where a patient has been harmed and compensation is being sought, the claimant may allege that a practitioner was at fault in failing to take proper care of the patient. At present in order to claim compensation, the claimant would have to establish that he was owed a duty of care, that there was a breach of this duty of care which has caused harm to the patient. This action is known as an action for negligence. An action for negligence is one of a group of civil actions known as 'torts' which can be brought in the civil courts for compensation to be paid.

Duty of care at work: the nurse owes a duty of care to her patients

Duty of care outside work: there is no duty recognised in law to volunteer assistance, however the NMC recognises that all practitioners have a professional duty at all times to provide assistance to others. (Clause 8.5 of the Code of Professional Conduct, NMC 2004)

Standards of care

The civil courts have used the Bolam Test to determine whether there is any negligence. This requires the reasonable standard of professionally approved practice to be followed. The Bolam Test was used in the case of Whitehouse v. Jordan where an obstetrician was alleged to have been negligent in delivering a baby by forceps:

> *When you get a situation that involves the use of some special skill or competence, then the test as to whether there has been negligence or not is . . . the standard of the ordinary skilled man exercising and professing to have that special skill. If a surgeon failed to measure up to that in any respect ('clinical judgement' or otherwise), he had been negligent and should be so adjudged.*

Evidence on what standard could have been expected in a given situation would be given to the courts by experts who would refer to research relating to clinically effective practice and to guidelines and recommendations of such bodies as the National Institute for Clinical Excellence, the Healthcare Commission and the National Service Frameworks and their appropriateness in relation to the actual circumstances of the case.

Clinical governance and standard setting

Section 18 of the Health Act 1999 imposed a duty upon NHS organisations to put into place and monitor quality standards. This is the foundation for the concept of clinical governance. Section 18 has been slightly amended by the Health and Social Care (Community Health and Standards) Act 2003 which has also given powers to the Secretary of State to publish standards which NHS organisations would have a duty to implement. The Department of Health has issued Standards for Better Health (DoH, 2004), which sets out the level of quality all organisations providing NHS care will be expected to meet.

Vicarious liability

An employer may be held liable where an employee has acted negligently or fraudulently in the course of employment. The consequences of this doctrine is that although the employee has been personally at fault, compensation is paid out by the employer to the victim. In theory the employer has a right to claim an indemnity from the negligent employee to re-compensate him. However this would rarely be exercised in the NHS.

Causation

Unless the claimant can establish that the harm which occurred was the result of the breach of the duty of care, compensation would not be payable. The harm must be a reasonably foreseeable consequence of the breach of duty.

Harm

Compensation is available for pain, suffering loss of amenity (eg the ability to walk, see etc) loss of earnings and death. Compensation is also paid for post traumatic stress disorder (Once called nervous shock) Loss or damage of property is also compensateable.

Future reforms

Because of the high cost of meeting claims for compensation for clinical negligence, the Department of Health issued a consultation paper (DoH, 2003) suggesting that a new scheme, to be called NHS Redress Scheme, should be introduced to provide a cheaper, speedier system of resolving disputes. At the time of writing, Government response to the feedback from the consultation is awaited.

Disciplinary action

Each employee has a contract with the employer which requires the employee to take reasonable care and to obey the reasonable instructions of the employer. Where there has been harm to a patient as a result of failings by the practitioner, the employer may institute disciplinary action which could lead to the dismissal of the employee. The employee may have the right to challenge this dismissal in the employment tribunal. New regulations require the employer to follow a strict code in hearing grievance disputes or taking disciplinary action.

Fitness to practise proceedings before the Nursing and Midwifery Council

Every practitioner registered with the NMC is required to follow the Code of Professional Conduct and if she has caused harm to a patient there would be a prima facie (at first sight) case that she was not fit to practice and therefore should not be on the register. Employers, police and members of the public report cases to the NMC who would investigate the case to decide if a hearing before one of its Practice Committees is required. The options open to the Conduct and Competence Committee if misconduct is found are:

1. Refer the matter to Screeners for mediation or itself undertake mediation.
2. Take no further action.
3. Striking off the Register:
4. Suspension for a specified period from the Register (not exceeding one year):
5. Impose conditions with which the person must comply for a specified period which shall not exceed three years (A conditions of practice order)

6. Caution the practitioner and make an order directing the Registrar to annotate the register accordingly for a specified period which shall not be for less than one year and not more than five years. (A caution order)
7. Refer to another Committee
8. Interim Orders

Patients' rights

Right to access care

The Secretary of State has a duty under NHS legislation to provide health services as far as he considers it necessary to meet all reasonable requirements. The courts have interpreted the statutory duty as limited and not giving patients an absolute right to have health services. Because of the mismatch between supply and demand the fact that a patient has to wait for services will not be actionable in court.

Right to consent

A mentally capacitated adult (ie someone over 18 years) has a right to consent to treatment or to refuse to give consent, even where the treatment is life saving. As long as the patient is mentally capable the refusal could be for a good reason, a bad reason or no reason at all. Treating a patient without consent is a trespass to the person and is actionable in the civil courts without proving that harm occurred. It may also be actionable in the criminal courts.
A mentally incapacitated adult, who is incapable of giving consent can be treated without consent, provided that the treatment is in his or her best interests and the Bolam Test of reasonable standard of care is followed. Relatives cannot give consent on behalf of a mentally incapacitated adult. Legislation to provide a statutory framework for decision making on behalf of a mentally incapacitated adult has been drafted and is at the time of writing being debated in Parliament. In Scotland there is the Adults with Incapacity (Scotland) Act 2000 which covers the situation.

Capacity

There is a presumption that a person over 16 years has the capacity to make decisions, but this presumption can be rebutted (removed) if there is evidence to the contrary. How is capacity determined?

The Court of Appeal has laid down the following test for incapacity:

A person lacks the capacity (to give a valid consent) if some impairment or disturbance of mental functioning renders the person unable to make a decision whether to consent to or to refuse treatment. That inability to make a decision will occur when:

a. The patient is unable to comprehend and retain the information which is material to the decision, especially as to the likely consequences of having or not having the treatment in question

b. The patient is unable to use the information and weigh it in the balance as part of the process of arriving at the decision

Children: young persons of 16 and 17 years

Young persons of 16 and 17 years have a statutory right to give consent to treatment, including medical dental and surgical and anaesthetic and diagnostic procedures under Section 8 Family Law Reform Act 1969. The refusal of a young person to life saving treatment will be overruled if the refusal is in the best interests of that person.

Children : below 16 years

The House of Lords decided in the Gillick case that in exceptional circumstances a child who had the requisite competence could give a valid consent to examination and treatment without parental involvement.

Parents

Parents have the right to give consent on behalf of their child up to the age of 18 years if that proposed treatment is in the best interests of the child. Where the child or young person is refusing treatment, the older the child, the less likely one would be to rely upon parental consent, and the more likely it would be to take the case to court which would determine what was in the best interests of the child. A declaration was sought from the court when a girl of 15 refused a heart transplant. The court made a declaration that a transplant was in her best interests.

In the event of a dispute between parents over significant treatment, an application to court would be made for a decision on what was in the best interests of the child to be determined under the Children Act 1989.

Parental responsibility

Where father and mother were married before the birth of the child, they retain parental responsibilities unless the child dies or is adopted or the court removes them. In all other cases the father must ensure that his name is on the birth certificate or he is recorded as having taken on parental responsibilities.

Guidance on consent

The Department of Health has published guidance on the law relating to consent and also forms which could be used to provide evidence that consent has been given (DoH, 2001). Form 4 can be used where a patient is incapable of giving consent. The Kennedy Report which followed the Inquiry into paediatric heart surgery in Bristol also made significant recommendations in relation to consent to treatment and the overall relationship between patient and professional.

Right to confidentiality

A duty to respect the confidentiality of patient information is binding on all health professionals and arises:

- from an implied duty in the contract of employment
- from the professional duty set out in the NMC code of professional conduct
- from the trust relationship which exists between patient and professional
- from specific statutory provisions such as the Data Protection Act 1998, the Human Rights Act 1998 Schedule 1 Article 8 of the European

Convention on Human Rights: the right to respect for private and family life and the Human Fertilisation and Embryology Acts 1990 and 1992.

Exceptions to this duty of confidentiality are recognised. Confidential information could be passed on:

- with the consent of the patient
- in the interests of the patient
- on the order of the court
- as a result of statutory provisions such as Public Health Acts, Road Traffic Acts, Prevention of Terrorism Acts
- in the public interest.

Disclosure in the public interest is recognised as an exception to the duty of confidentiality by the NMC. Clause 5.3 states that disclosures can be made where:

they can be justified in the public interest (usually where disclosure is essential to protect the patient or client or someone else from the risk of significant harm).

Good practice would ensure that a record is kept of the disclosure and the justification for it.

Right to access health records

Under statutory instruments published under powers set out in the Data Protection Act 1998 a patient can access his health records except in the following situations:

- Where the access 'would be likely to cause serious harm to the physical or mental health or condition of the data subject or any other person (which may include a health professional).'
- Where a third party (not being a health professional caring for the patient) has asked not to be identified and access to that part of the record would identify the individual.

Right to complain

Every patient has a right to complain and new organisations have been established to facilitate this and support the patient. They include:

- Commission for Patient and Public Involvement in Health
- Independent Complaints and Advice Service (ICAS)
- Patient advice and liaison service (PALS)

Further information can be obtained from the Department of Health website. Regulations have been introduced to set up a new complaints procedure. There are three stages:

- Local investigation and response to the complaint
- Independent review conducted by the Healthcare Commission
- Health Service Commissioner (Ombudsman) or Local Authority Commissioner

Conclusions

These are only a few of the main areas of law which apply to health care practitioners. Others are covered in chapters of this book: health and safety law and the law relating to medicines. Other topics such as the law on mental health, law relating to death, personal property, and specialist areas of practice can be found in the author's books listed below. New statutes regulations and cases may change what has been written here and practitioners should endeavour, as in other areas of their practice, to keep up to date.

References

Department of Health (2001) Reference Guide to Consent for Examination or Treatment DH 2001; www. doh.gov.uk/consent; Department of Health good practice in consent implementation guide November 2001. DH

Department of Health (June 2003) Making Amends A consultation paper setting out proposals for reforming the approach to clinical negligence in the NHS. CMO

Department of Health (2004) National Standards, Local Action, Health and socail Care Standards and Planning Framework (incorporates Standards for Better Health as Appendix A) July. London

Dimond B (2004) The Legal Aspects of Nursing, 4th edition. Pearson Education. London

F. v. West Berkshire Health Authority [1989] 2 All ER 545; [1990] 2 AC 1

Gillick v. West Norfolk and Wisbech AHA and the DHSS 1985 3 All ER 402
R. v. Adomako [1995] 1 AC 171; [1994] 3 All ER 79
R. v. Secretary of State for Social Services ex parte Hincks and others, Solicitors' Journal 29 June 1979 436
Re MB (Adult Medical Treatment) [1997] 2 FLR 426
Whitehouse v. Jordan [1981] 1 All ER 267
Re W (a minor) (medical treatment) 1992 4 All ER 627
Re M (Medical Treatment Consent) [1999] 2 FLR 1097
Bristol Royal Infirmary Inquiry (Kennedy Report) Learning from Bristol: the report of the public inquiry into children's heart surgery at the Bristol Royal Infirmary 1984-1995 Command paper CM 5207 Stationery Office London 2001
Nursing and Midwifery Council (2004) Code of Professional Conduct: Standards for Conduct, Performance and Ethics. NCM, London

Additional reading

Dimond BC (2004) Legal Aspects of Nursing. 4th edition, Pearson Education, London
Dimond BC (2002) Legal Aspects of Midwifery. 2nd edition, Books for Midwives Press
Dimond BC (2003)Legal Aspects of Consent. Quay Publications Mark Allen Press, Dinton Salisbury
Dimond BC (2002) Legal Aspects of Patient Confidentiality. Quay Publications Mark Allen Press, Dinton Salisbury
Dimond BC (2002) Legal Aspects of Pain Management. Quay Publications Mark Allen Press. Dinton Salisbury
Kennedy I and Grubb A (2000) Medical Law. 3rd edition. Butterworth, London
McHale J and Tingle J (2001) Law and Nursing. Butterworth Heineman London
Stauch M, Wheat K and Tingle J (2002) Source Book on Medical Law, 2nd edition, Cavendish Publishing, London

Useful websites.

www.nelh.gov.uk/consent
www.dh.gov.uk/modernisationboardreport/index.htm
www.dh.gov.uk/nhsfoundationtrusts/independentregulator.htm
www.the-shipman-inquiry.org.uk/reports.asp
www.bristol-inquiry.org.uk

Chapter 21

Professional nursing and midwifery practice

George Castledine

The Nursing and Midwifery Council (NMC) is the regulatory body for nursing, midwifery and health visiting. It was set up in 1998 following a governmental review of the legislation governing the United Kingdom Central Council (UKCC) and the National Nursing Boards for England, Scotland, Wales and Northern Ireland.

Background

The purpose of any governmental regulation of professional clinical practice, including nursing, is the protection of the public's health, safety and welfare. Professions or occupations where there is a potential risk of harm to the consumer are always under scrutiny and consideration for regulation. In the past nursing like medicine was given the freedom of self-regulation but due to the demands for more public involvement, the regulation of nursing has changed. There is now greater public participation in all the healthcare professions.

The key tasks of the NMC are to:

• maintain a register of qualified nurses, midwives and health visitors
• set standards for nursing, midwifery and health visiting education, practice and conduct
• provide advice for nurses on professional standards
• consider allegations of misconduct or unfitness to practice due to ill health.

The paramount consideration of the regulatory process is to ensure public safety through safe and effective practice of nursing. All practising nurses, whatever their field, have to be registered with the Council.

Professional conduct

The NMC investigates complaints against registered nurses, midwives and health visitors about professional misconduct or unfitness to practice. Anyone can make a complaint about a nurse's behaviour. The most common sources are employers and the police.

The types of misconduct which could lead to removal from the register include:

* physically or verbally abusing patients
* stealing from patients
* failing to care for patients' property
* failing to document and keep appropriate nursing records
* committing serious criminal offences
* dealing in or abusing drugs.

The NMC only deals with misconduct which, if proved, would be serious enough to justify removing a practitioner's name from the register. Allegations of misconduct have to be proved therefore it is important to weigh up the evidence before reporting someone.

Reporting a case to the NMC

The following information will be required if a case if referred to the council:

* the practitioners full name, PIN and most recent address
* a description of the practitioner's job at the time of the alleged misconduct
* a description of the workplace, including the numbers and types of clients for whom the practitioner was responsible
* a description of staff numbers, grades and reporting lines at the workplace
* an account of the alleged misconduct
* copies of any witness statements
* copies of any relevant documents such as care plans, drug charts and work diaries
* copies of management notes of any investigative or disciplinary meetings
* details of any police involvement
* details of practitioner's previous job
* details of any relevant training and education since qualifying
* details of any previous disciplinary action or counselling.

Interim suspension of registration

In exceptional cases the NMC can suspend a practitioner's registration before the case is fully investigated and goes through the system.

The preliminary proceedings committee usually sorts out the serious cases for further action and also deals with interim suspension. It can only consider this when there is some evidence of continuing serious risk, either to patients or the practitioner themselves.

The health committee

When health is an issue or the cause of a practitioner being unfit to practice, it may be appropriate to refer them to the NMC's health committee. The committee can either suspend or remove ill practitioners following health assessment and evidence of the practitioner being a risk to patients or themselves.

Examples of conditions that might seriously impair a practitioner's fitness to practice:

- alcohol dependency
- drug dependency
- untreated serious mental health
- serious personality disorder
- a chronic illness which has gone untreated
- severe effects of stress
- physical ill health due to family or social problems.

Reporting a case to the health committee

If you report a case to the health committee, a statutory declaration form has to be signed and submitted to the committee. It will also need:

- the practitioners full name, PIN and most recent address
- details of the practitioner's sickness record and copies of any medical reports
- an account of any behaviour which shows unfitness to practice
- copies of witness statements about any such behaviour or incidents
- copies of any management notes of any hearings where the practitioner's fitness to practice has been discussed.

The Code of Professional Conduct

The NMC Code of Professional Conduct is used as the benchmark for judging professional misconduct. The latest version was published in 2004 and is divided into eight sections covering:

- respect for the patient or client as an individual
- protection and support for patients
- behaviour that justifies the trust and confidence of the public
- duty to care for patients
- upholding and enhancing the good reputation of the profession
- obtaining consent before giving treatments and/or nursing care
- protection of confidential information
- co-operation with others in the team
- maintenance of professional knowledge and competence
- being trustworthy
- action to identify and minimise risks to patients and clients.

Figure 21.1 The process of professional conduct

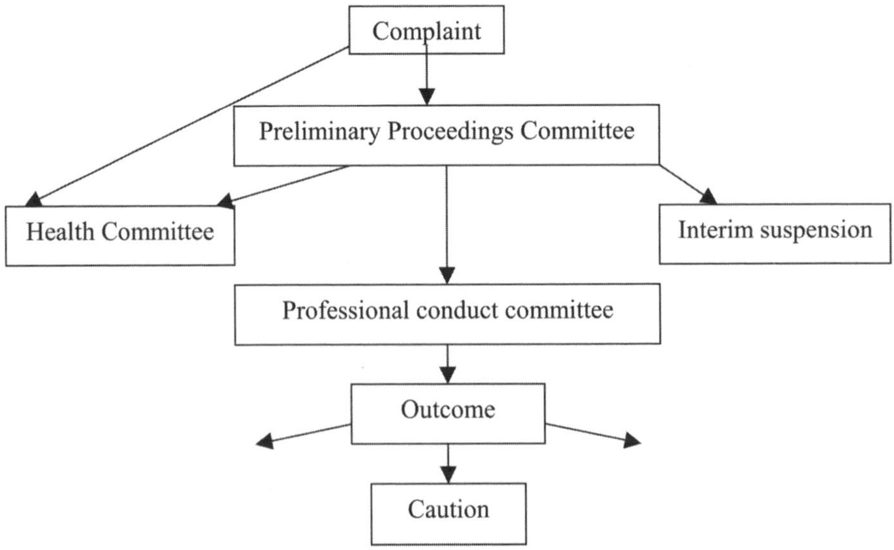

Approximately 100 practitioners are removed from the register every year. Over 50 are cautioned, which means that although misconduct was proved there is reasonable mitigation and the person is not a risk to the public. A record of caution is kept on the practitioner's file for five years.

Practice-related offences

The following are common types of practice-related offences that lead to professional conduct hearings:

- physical/verbal abuse of patients
- failure/inappropriate attention to basic needs and the fundamentals/essence of care
- failure to keep accurate records or report incidents
- unsafe clinical practice
- sexual harassment or bullying
- drug related incidents
- dishonesty or theft
- sexual abuse of patients/clients
- misadministration of drugs
- failures in communication.

Sphere of practice

The following are areas in which many offences occur:

- offences not related to work but could lead to unfitness to practise eg. violence, sexual offences, dealing or importing drugs
- nursing home
- care of the elderly
- medical/ surgical nursing
- mental health nursing
- community nursing
- midwifery
- accident and emergency
- management
- paediatrics.

Case history

A nurse who did not keep accurate fluid balance records and was rude

Monitoring a patient's fluid balance is a serious business which on many general wards is carried out in a haphazard and inaccurate way. Too many patients are placed on fluid balance charts who do not really need their intake and output monitoring closely. This leads to careless practice and sends out a message that fluid monitoring is not as important as it should be.

In the following case, a ward at a large teaching hospital in London held the view that fluid balance charts, if present, should be completed as correctly as possible. Jean, the ward manager, was always emphasising this point and the staff introductory pack to the ward clearly spelt out this message to new staff and students.

Rachel had qualified as a staff nurse two years previously and had worked in a variety of clinical settings. When she arrived on Jean's ward she received the usual inducation programme, including the need for accuracy in fluid balance monitoring.

Soon after, one of the senior nurses noticed that Rachel was very poor at recording actual amounts which the patients had received by mouth. She would often put down that a patient had received a full glass of water or a cup of tea when in fact this was not true. It seemed that Rachel assumed that patients had drunk everything she placed before them. The senior staff nurse discussed this with Rachel, who agreed that she was a bit neglectful and would improve her recording.

Several months later, a patient who had been in the intensive care unit and had been receiving strict measurement of her fluid balance because of renal problems was transferred to the ward. When Jean made her evening round following Rachel's shift she was approached by the patient's relatives. They were very concerned about the way Rachel had behaved. Rachel had insisted that the patient use a bedpan in bed when it had previously been much easier for her to use a commode. Further, when the patient asked if she could wash her hands, she had been told to wait until after visiting time. Finally, because the patient had experienced difficulties using the bedpan, the bed was wet and Rachel had shouted at the patient in full hearing of the ward.

Jean reassured the relatives and spoke to the patient about the incident. It seemed that Rachel had said to the patient that because she had wet the bed it had ruined the fluid balance and that this would result in problems in medical treatment. When Jean checked the fluid balance charts of all Rachel's patients, she found that there were some major errors and omissions.

Rachel was very angry when Jean spoke to her the next day and said that she was not the only person on the ward who failed to keep the fluid balance charts up to date. She also stated that Jean's ward was 'too obsessed' with fluid balance and other wards in the hospital were much more easy to work on. Rachel was suspended from duty because the patient made an official complaint about her behaviour.

Rachel refused to co-operate with the enquiry and left the trust without informing it of her new address. It was therefore decided to refer her case to the NMC, but Rachel also declined to co-operate with the NMC investigation. She was found guilty by a professional conduct committee of three charges, two relating to her poor fluid balance recording and one charge of speaking and dealing inappropriately with a patient when she wanted to use a commode. Her name was removed from the register.

Castledine (2003)

Breach of the Code of Professional Conduct

In this case, the following clauses of the Code are relevant:

- **1.4:** You have a duty of care for your patients and clients, who are entitled to receive safe and competent care
- **2.1:** You must recognise and respect the role of patients and clients as partners in their care and the contribution they can make to it. This involves identifying their preferences regarding care and respecting these with the limits of professional practice, exisiting legislation, resources and the goals of the therapeutic relationship.
- **2.2:** You are personally accountable for ensuring that you promote and protect the interest and dignity of patients and clients, irrespective of gender, age, race, ability, sexuality, economic status, lifestyle, culture, religious or political belief.
- **4.7:** You have a duty to co-operate with internal and external investigations.

Post registration education and practice (PREP)

The PREP requirements are professional standards set by the NMC. They are legal requirements which all nurses must meet in order to renew their registration.

There are two separate PREP standards that affect a nurse's registration:

1. The PREP (Practice) standard: The nurse must have worked in some capacity by virtue of their nursing qualification during the previous five years a minimum of 100days (750 hours) or have successfully undertaken an approved return to practice course.
2. The PREP (continuing professional development) standard: The nurse must have undertaken and recorded their continuing professional development over the three years prior to renewal of registration.
   - You should have undertaken at least five days or thirty-five hours of learning activity relevant to their practice during the three years prior to their renewal of registration.
   - You should have maintained a personal, professional profile of their learning activity .
   - You should comply with any request from the NMC to audit how they have met these requirements.

Keeping a personal professional profile (PPP)

The way in which CPD can be recorded is clarified by the NMC in its PREP handbook (NMC, 2002). This states that the standard involves the maintenance of a PPP of a nurse's learning activity. Although there is no such thing as an approved PREP/CPD learning activity, all nurses must document in a PPP relevant learning and the way in which it has informed and influenced their practice.

There is no officially approved format for the PPP but the NMC does outline a simple template that the nurse might like to consider. This design is included in the PREP handbook. Chapter 23 also offers an outline. The NMC handbook also contains examples of how various nurses working in a variety of settings and specialties have described their learning activity, the outcomes and the way this has influenced them in their work. This fairly simple procedure forms the basis of what every nurse's PPP should be about and is the bare minimum of what is expected of every registered nurse in the UK.

What has happened, however, is that the proposed content of profiles has been hijacked by over enthusiastic educationalists and others who have, in many cases, exaggerated what should be included in such documents.

A profile could easily be stored on a computer with a back-up-disc; it does not have to be in paper form. However, it is suggested that a profile should be contained in a large clip folder and be divided into three main sections.

- **The first section:** should contain personal information about yourself and a CV which follows a chronological order so that you can easily use the information for a job application in the future.

- **The second section:** should be the core education and training information required by the NMC for re-registration purposes. This should include a detailed record of your continuing formal and informal education ie. organised courses and study days plus any other learning activity that has influenced your work.
- **The third section:** should include reflections on critical incidents which have occurred in practice and may well service as learning experiences for the future.

This simple approach to keeping a PPP is all that is required. It helps nurses to recognise and record their achievements, assist in personal planning and development, and reflect carefully and evaluate their experiences, thus encouraging accountability. Critical factors in keeping a profile are: good self-discipline, ability to reflect and record experiences, flexibility and easy accessibility to a system that is simple, straightforward, precise and concise.

Continued competency in hospital nursing

Hospital nursing practice is becoming more complex and demanding. There is now a need to keep up to date with the extensive and increasing amount of scientific information, governmental reports and proposals. Failure to maintain standards of practice could lead to an increase in errors, increased risk of patient harm and a lack of public confidence. The NMC is carefully looking at ways to measure and ensure nurses maintain their competency for the role they are in. Evidence from the increasing number of cases submitted to the NMC that constitute perceived incompetence in practice is a major concern and serves as a timely reminder to all nurses to pursue continuing education and lifelong learning.

Competence means the integration of the professional attributes required for the performance of the scope of nursing in a given role or situation and in accordance with the standards of practice.

Professional attributes means knowledge, skills, judgement, self concept (attitudes and values), trait and motives

(Campbell 1998)

Scope of practice

The scope of practice was introduced by the UKCC in 1992 and is widely accepted as referring to those changing aspects of healthcare that can be integrated into a nurse's role without detriment to the purpose, function and safety of that individual's care.

Scope of practice is intended to encourage dynamic nursing practice and integrate certain skills and medical tasks which the nurse feels will enable them to deliver more efficient, sensitive holistic nursing. What it is not trying to encourage is a shift into medicine or a more medical role for nurses. The scope of practice is not there to put patients at risk, or to encourage nurses to do what they fancy and pick up medical tasks which are of interest to them. It is important that the nurse is given adequate education and training before carrying out such developments. A nurse should never forget the importance of carrying out and properly supervising the fundamental and core aspects of nursing (see *chapter 17*).

The NMC's main purpose is to establish and improve standards for the nursing profession in order to serve and protect the public. It regularly produces reports and guidelines some of which are listed below in the section on additional reading.

Remember what you can do

- Make sure you re-register every three years.
- Keep up to date with the Professional Code of Conduct and remember your responsibilities regarding this.
- Discuss with senior nurses or the Nursing director concerns you may have about issues of misconduct or concerns about a practitioner's health.
- Ask for update sessions and discussions on the Code of Conduct.
- Keep up to date with education, training and practice to meet the PREP standards.
- Keep a personal professional profile and ensure it is up to date.
- Heed the advice of the NMC and carefully take notice of any new proposals it makes.

References

Campbell B (1998) Consultation Report on Competence Assessment. College of Nurses. Ontario, Canada

Castledine G (2003) Nurse who did not keep accurate fluid balance records and was rude. Professional Misconduct Case 95: Fluid balance recording. *Br J Nurs* **12**(12): 717

Nursing and Midwifery Council (2004) The Prep Handbook. NMC, London

Nursing and Midwifery Council (2004) Code of Professional Conduct. NMC, London

Additional reading

Guidelines for the administration of medicines (2004)

Annual Reports on Professional Conduct

Supporting nurses and midwives through lifelong learning (2002)

The PREP handbook (2004)

Practitioner–client relationships and the prevention of abuse (2002)

Guidelines for records and record keeping (2005)

Copies of all above NMC Publications are available from:

NMC Publications, 23Portland Place. London W1B 1P2
Email: publications@nmc-uk.org

NMC Professional advice service, 23 Portland Place, London W1B 1PZ
Tel: 020 7333 6541/6550/6553
Fax: 020 7333 6538
Email: advice@nmc-uk.org

Davies C, Beach A (2000) Interpreting Professional self-regulation. Routledge, London

Useful websites

www.nmc-uk.org   Nursing and Midwifery Council

www.modern.nhs.uk   Modernisation Agency

Chapter 22

Clinical support

Ann Close

No one would argue with the premise that the NHS is rapidly changing in its efforts to modernise. Development and support are becoming increasingly important in helping nurses and midwives cope with the changes in their working environment and continue to be safe and effective practitioners. As a result, a number of support mechanisms have been developed including preceptorship, mentorship, clinical supervision, and practice-based education as well as more general support. These are relevant to nurses at all levels from students, to nurses returning to practice, from newly registered to experienced practitioners. Although there are differences in these forms of support, in reality there is confusion and sometimes the terms are used interchangeably. This chapter attempts to provide some clarity in the types of support available and highlights the benefits and factors to consider when using any of the clinical support mechanisms.

Preceptorship

The concept of a preceptor was formally introduced by the UKCC in 1993 (UKCC 1993). This was in response to a realisation that Project 2000 (1986) qualified nurses needed a period of support to help them move from a being a supernumerary student to becoming an accountable registered nurse. The Council's policy was that all newly registered nurses, midwives and health visitors should be provided with a period of support for approximately the first four months as a registered practitioner. They also felt that practitioners returning to practice after a break of five or more years should equally be given such support. Morton-Cooper and Palmer (1993) define a preceptor as:

> *... a qualified and experienced first level nurse who has agreed to work in partnership with a newly registered practitioner colleague in order to assist and support them in the process of learning and adaptation to his or her role.*

According to the UKCC (1993) preceptors should:

- Have sufficient knowledge of the practitioner's programme to identify current learning needs.
- Help the practitioner to apply knowledge to practice.
- Understand how practitioners integrate into a new practice setting and assist them in this process.
- Understand and assist with the problems of transition from pre-registration student to registered and accountable practitioner.
- Set, with the practitioner, objectives for learning to assist with this transition.

At the end of the period the practitioner should be ready to assume primary practice in the opinion of the practitioner and the preceptor. Some organisations have expanded the scope of preceptorship to include any clinical nurse undergoing role transition.

Mentorship

Mentoring is also concerned with helping individuals in their development but is often used to describe a longer term relationship. Morton-Cooper and Palmer (1993) define a mentor as:

> *... someone who provides an enabling relationship which facilitates another's growth and development.*

Mentorship is concerned with promoting personal change by helping another:

- understand and learn from day-to-day experiences
- develop confidence
- develop creativity and innovation
- become more self aware
- take calculated risks
- fulfil their potential
- develop and advance their careers.

A mentor achieves this through:

- Challenging the individual: encouraging them to confront their beliefs and values, presenting them with conflicts for resolution and offering new ideas and new ways of doing things for them to consider. This may include setting tasks and targets.

- Support: through listening to concerns, providing encouragement when things are getting difficult, sharing own experiences and celebrating successes.
- Sponsorship: helping individuals open doors to new experiences and opportunities which will help them achieve their potential and lead to career advancement.

Clinical supervision

Although clinical supervision has been in practice for many years it has only become high on the nursing agenda for the past 10 years. It was first promoted in the nursing, midwifery and health visiting strategy Vision for the Future (NHS Management Executive, 1993). Since then the importance of supervision in assisting individuals to learn from their experiences to aid personal development and effectiveness has been highlighted and encouraged in national strategies and documents (UKCC, 1996, DoH, 1998a, 1998b & 1999).

There are many definitions which describe the process of supervision which provides a formal mechanism for discussing practice and work related situations.

The 1993 Vision for the Future described it as:

a formal process of professional support and learning which enables individual nurses to develop knowledge and competence, assume responsibility for their practice and enhance consumer protection and the safety of care in a complex situation.

(NHS Management Executive, 1993)

The UKCC issued a position statement on clinical supervision in 1996 in which it stated that clinical supervision:

brings practitioners and skilled supervisors together to reflect on practice. Supervision aims to identify solutions to problems, improve practice and increase understanding of professional issues.

(UKCC, 1996)

There are a number of models of supervision. Proctor (1991) suggests there are three functions.

- The normative or management function: which is about quality control and ensuring policies and procedures are understood and followed and standards are developed, followed and audited.
- The restorative function or pastoral support: which provides support to enable practitioners to understand and manage the emotional stress of nursing practice.
- The formative or education function: which is involved with the educational process of developing skills, ability and knowledge to assist in delivering evidence-based practice.

Reflection is also an important function of supervision. Schon (1987) described two types of reflection which are used in clinical supervision.

- Reflection in action: occurs when the individual reflects on their experience as it is occurring and while they are practising in the clinical area. It can influence the decisions they make and the care given in their immediate situation.
- Reflection on action: this involves looking back on incidents that have occurred. Critical incidents or other events that have happened are considered and the supervisee with the supervisors support, analyses these to determine what was handled well and what could have been done differently the next time.

Delivery of clinical supervision

This may be achieved through one-to one supervision or group supervision. The advantages and disadvantages can be seen below. (Table 22.1)

Table 22.1 Advantages and disadvantages of group v one-to-one supervision		
	Advantages	Disadvantages
One to one supervision	– Individualised attention – Easier to arrange supervision sessions	– Learning is limited to the experiences of the supervisor and supervisee – Process is only as effective as the supervisor's ability
Group supervision	– Learning from a range of other people – More cost effective in terms of supervisor time – Wider dissemination of good practice	– Sometimes difficult to ensure all group are available to attend supervision – Reluctance to raise some issues in group situation

Practice-based education

Many practitioners relate teaching in the clinical setting to pre-registration students but teaching in the clinical setting is just as relevant to registered nurses and midwives and is carried out in different ways.

- Clinical teaching rounds: Discussion of patients and their care is undertaken in the clinical setting or it may involve demonstrations of care by a more experienced practitioner.
- Planned teaching sessions: A rolling programme may be developed for the staff on a range of clinical topics, professional issues and management issues. Staff may be expected to lead one of the sessions.
- Demonstration and supervised practice: This may be done on a formal or informal basis where a more experienced member of staff demonstrates a procedure and then supervises and assesses others.
- Role models: This occurs when a nurse observes another's behaviour, identifies with it and tries to emulate it. It is important that the behaviour displayed is seen as desirable, that the nurse is capable of learning the behaviour and that the role model points out the essential cues.
- Practice Development Nurses: Many departments or specialties have established specific posts to help them develop practices, new ways of working and enhance the knowledge and skills of staff. This may be achieved through many of the above and also through
  - one to one situations, where the nurse pairs with the practice development nurse to carry out care
  - research evaluation and audit to develop and test out new ways of working.

Stress management

Chapter 11 has already highlighted that work-related stress is on the increase. Although it is recognised that employers have an obligation to identify and manage factors causing stress, employees too have a role to play.

You should be aware of:

- Factors in your working environment: These include increased work demands, role conflict and ambiguity, management and leadership style, harassment and bullying behaviour by others, lack of control, anxiety about changes planned or career prospects, poor physical environment and many more. Traumatic incidents can also have prolonged effects leading to stress.

- Personal factors: These include unreliable childcare arrangements, relationship or financial problems, illness, bereavement, house moves among others.
- The effects of stress: These include physical effects such as high blood pressure, headaches, nausea, lethargy, repeated infections, ulcers, anxiety, depression and behavioural changes including sleep disturbances, lapses in concentration, impairment of memory and judgement, indecisiveness, changes in eating habits, increase in smoking and alcohol intake and irritability.
- Ways you can help yourself
  - find out if your Trust has a policy or guidance on stress management and what there is on offer. This might include stress management courses, assertiveness training and information on where you can get additional help
  - try to keep a healthy balance between work and leisure. Make sure you spend time on your interests
  - consider discussing your views with your line manager and negotiating alternatives, such as different ways of working, or changes to your hours of work
  - discuss strategies for managing stress with your mentor or during clinical supervision sessions.
- Where you can get help:
  - find out if your hospital provides
  1. an occupational health service, they should be able to provide access to counselling services or make referrals to specialist doctors or nurses if there is an underlying medical problem
  2. a confidential staff counselling facility
  3. a 'whistle blowing' policy, and other policies which indicate what action you can take such as those on 'handling violence and aggression', or 'management of harassment and bullying'.
  - hospital chaplains often take a lead in helping staff deal with stress
  - Citizens Advice Bureaus can provide financial advice and information on organisations that can help with relationship problems such as Relate
  - your family and friends
  - your GP.

Requirements for clinical support

- Policies and guidelines: These will be necessary to ensure a consistent and standardised approach across an organisation. This will create a feeling of fairness and will also be helpful if individuals move within the organisation. The policy should be sufficiently flexible to adapt to the specific needs of the ward or department.
- Preparation of staff: It is essential that individuals undertaking clinical support are prepared appropriately for the role and that they have the necessary background experience.
- Confidentiality: Agreements of the ground rules must be agreed by all parties and adhered to otherwise trust will be lost and the support mechanisms will break down.
- Operation within the code of professional conduct: Actions that will be taken in the event of a nurse's negligence, misconduct or incompetence should also be made clear in the policies and the person responsible for taking this action should be identified. There should be recognition that, as registered nurses, each individual is accountable for their practice.
- Documentation: Agreements about how the content, outcomes and action plans of the support are recorded, who has access to these records and where they are stored must be agreed.
- Links to management systems: Clinical support should be seen as an adjunct to management and teaching and as an important part of clinical governance as it helps to maintain and improve standards of care.
- Choice of supervisor: Individuals should, where possible, have a choice of who provides clinical support. Trust and respect are essential, although this shouldn't become a 'cosy' arrangement.
- Management commitment: Managers must be committed to clinical support and provide essential resources to develop and implement systems.

Benefits of clinical support

All of the mechanisms for clinical support have similar benefits including:

- Improved patient care – skills and knowledge develop as a result of reflecting on practice in real life situations.
- Dissemination of good practice – sharing experiences helps others learn.

- Increased confidence – examining and discussing practice will help nurses articulate and give a rationale for what they are doing. They will also cope more easily with difficulties and problems.
- Improved performance – by examining practice, nurses can develop ways of working more effectively rather than just working harder.
- Increased job satisfaction – any form of clinical support suggests to the individual that they are worth investing time and effort on and that they are an important part of the team. This will help them to be more motivated and enthusiastic about their work.
- Reduced risks in practice – by looking at different, safer and better ways of doing things.
- Identification of training, development needs and priorities – provides the opportunity for individuals to identify their strengths and weaknesses.
- Helping an individual cope with the stresses of work and directing them to coping strategies or additional support.
- Developing staff and preparing them for career progression.

Barriers to effective clinical support

- May be seen by individuals and their managers as a burden – another task to complete.
- Concerns that it may reveal individual or collective shortcomings.
- Lack of appropriate venues near the workplace.
- Finding time for supervision due to other competing priorities.
- Perception that clinical support is managerial surveillance.

Remember what you can do

- Find out what clinical support mechanisms are available in your organisation. Ask your line manager or senior nurse.
- Read the relevant policies and guidelines for your organisation.
- Read more about the support mechanisms in journal articles and books.
- Find out what training opportunities there are to develop more understanding and the necessary skills.
- Ask colleagues what it is like in practice.

- Think how you can support others in your team and develop practices.
- Consider what clinical teaching you can offer in your clinical area.
- Identify positive role models in your experience and identify what positive characteristics and behaviours you can adopt.
- Make sure you are aware of the effects of stress for yourself and others.
- Find out what help is available to you.
- Don't forget senior colleagues need support too.

References

Department of Health (1998a) A First Class Service; Quality in the new NHS. NHS Executive, Leeds

Department of Health (1998b) The New NHS:Working Together: Securing a Quality Workforce for the NHS. HMSO, London

Department of Health (1999) The New NHS, Modern Dependable. HMSO, London

Morton-Cooper A, Palmer A (1993) Mentoring and Preceptorship – A Guide to Support Roles in Clinical Practice. Blackwell Scientific Publications, London

NHS Management Executive (1993) A Vision for the Future: The Nursing, Midwifery and Health Visiting Contribution to Health and Health Care. DoH, London

Proctor B (1991) On being a trainer and supervision for counselling in action. In: Butterworth A, Faugier J (1995) Clinical Supervision in Nursing, Midwifery and Health Visiting. A briefing paper. Manchester University

Schon D (1987) The reflective practitioner In: Minghella E, Benson A (1995) Developing reflective practice in mental health nursing through clinical incident analysis. *J Adv Nurs* 21: 205–13

United Kingdom Central Council for Nursing, Midwifery and Health Visiting (1993) Registrar's Letter The Council's Position Concerning a Period of Support and Preceptorship: Implementation of the Psot registration Education and Practice Project proposals. January 4 UKCC, London

United Kingdom Central Council for Nursing, Midwifery and Health Visiting (1996) Position Statement on clinical supervision and Health Visiting. UKCC, London

United Kingdom Central Council for Nursing, Midwifery and Health Visiting (1986) Project 2000: A New Preparation for Practice. UKCC, London

Additional reading

Amos D (2001) An evaluation of staff nurse role transition. *Nurs Standard* **16**(3): 36–41

Bowles N, Young C (1999) An evaluation study of clinical supervision based on Proctor's three function interactive model. *J Adv Nurs* **30**(4): 958–64

Butterworth T, Faugier J (1992) Clinical Supervision and Mentorship in Nursing. Chapman & Hall, London

Evans K (2001) Expectations of newly qualified nurses. *Nurs Standard* **15**(4:) 33–8

Fawcett D (2002) Mentoring – what it is and how to make it work. *AORN* **75**(5): 950–4

Howatson-Jones IL (2003) Difficulties in supervision and lifelong learning. *Nurs Standard* **17**(37): 37–41

Hyrkäs K, AppelQuist-Schmidlechner K (2003) Team supervision in multiprofessional teams: team members' descriptions of the effects as highlighted by group interviews. *J Clin Nurs* **12**(2): 188–97

Jones Alun (1998) Getting going with clinical supervision: an introductory seminar. *J Adv Nurs* **27**(3): 560–6

Kelly D, Simpson S, Brown P (2002) An action research project to evaluate the clinical practice facilitator roles for junior nurses in an acute hospital setting. *J Clin Nurs* **11**(1): 90–8

Spouse J (2001) Bridging theory and practice in the supervisory relationship: a sociocultural perspective. *J Adv Nurs* **33**(4): 512–22

Winstanley J, White E (2003). Clinical Supervision: models, measures, best practice. *Nurs Res* **10**(4): 7–38

Useful websites

www.nelh.org.uk	National Electronic Library for Health
www.rcn.org.uk	Royal College of Nursing
www.nursing-standard.co.uk	Nursing Standard
www.dh.gov.uk	Department of Health

Chapter 23
Continuing professional development

Ann Close

This chapter describes the benefits of continuing professional development (CPD) and how you can take responsibility by developing your portfolio, making the best use of your appraisal and making the most of all the opportunities you come across.

What is CPD and why is it necessary?

The majority of people including nurses go to work and want to do a good job. Healthcare and, therefore, nursing is rapidly changing, there are new technologies, developments in policy and practice as a result of research and new ways of working to improve access to and the quality of care. This requires nurses not only to develop new knowledge and skills, but also to keep existing skills and knowledge up to date. Continuing professional development is about harnessing opportunities that will enable nurses to do this.

How do I get started?

The following points will be helpful for any nurse whether they are looking for a high flying career in nursing or wish to develop in their current role.

Portfolio

The building blocks are your profile and portfolio. These describe you and your career history to date and can be divided into five main sections as shown in Table 23.1. It is essential that it is kept up to date not only for professional registration reasons but for developing your career.

Table 23.1: Sections for portfolio development

Personal Information	Name Date of birth Address Telephone numbers Registration details	Cultural background Characteristics Values and principles Strengths and weaknesses Significant roles in life	Coping mechanisms Interests Leisure activities Life experiences Health record
General education	Secondary education Qualifications obtained Subjects Awarding body Level/Grade/Year Personal achievements Key responsibilities	Further education College attended Number of years Qualifications Subjects Awarding body Level/grade/year Personal achievements Key responsibilities	Higher education Name of institution Number of years Qualifications Subjects Awarding body Level/grade/year Personal achievements Key responsibilities

Professional
education
	Recognised course
	    leading to
	    qualification
		Recognised study days
		    or short courses and
		    conferences attended
			Other professional
			    developments
			    – type and content
			    and application to
			    practice

Employment	Previous employment
	Employer.
	Date commenced.
	Date finished.
	Responsibilities of
	    post.
	Achievements.
	Transferable skills.
	Reasons for leaving
		Current employment
		Type of post and grade
		Employing authority
		Date commenced
		Responsibilities
		Personal and professional
		    development
		Additional roles
		Achievements
			Past and current
			    voluntary work
			Details and
			    responsibilities

Reflections on
practice
	Significant events
	    affecting practice
	Description of events.
	By whom were they
	    handled.
	Learning from events.
	Outcomes.
	Lessons learned
		Research projects
		Title
		Date completed
		Research role
		Reasons for undertaking
		    research /project
		Application to practice
			Publications
			    conference papers
			Reference of
			    publication
			Abstract of article

Start as you mean to go on

During your pre-registration training you will have combined academic study with clinical practice. It will help if you can continue to do this.

Many organisations offer staff nurse development programmes for newly registered nurses. This is worthwhile if you have the opportunity as it will help you consolidate learning from pre-registration training and develop into your new role as a staff nurse.

Preceptorship support is a requirement for newly registered nurses. It is intended to enable practitioners to develop their knowledge and skills with more experienced colleagues during the period of transition, usually for the first six months (*chapter 22*).

These are good starting points in your first year and they can be built on with the following.

Using appraisal, self-appraisal and personal development planning

Appraisal and self-appraisal

The aim of an appraisal system is to give each individual the opportunity to spend time with their manager and review their performance in their role, consider how it may develop in future and what opportunities, experiences and support are needed to do this. There are different formats for appraisal – some use competencies and others objectives or there may be a combination of both. With the introduction of Agenda for Change these will also have to include the Knowledge and Skills Framework (KSF). It is important that both the individual and manager prepares for the appraisal.

The individual should undertake a self-assessment and:

- Check progress against objectives, knowledge and skills outlines or competencies and determine if these are still appropriate to your role.
- Check your current job description and identify if you have taken up any additional roles and responsibilities.
- Identify your major achievements in the last 12 months.
- Identify areas of your role you think you are performing well.
- Identify if there are areas where you need further development and support.
- Consider whether you believe the best is being made of your skills and abilities.
- Consider where you want to go in career terms.

It is important to use your portfolio and reflective diary to help you in this self-assessment and provide you with evidence of your performance.

The manager should prepare for the appraisal by:

- Considering your performance over the last twelve months, highlighting achievements and disappointments.
- Considering whether your skills and abilities are being used to the best advantage.
- Identifying any specific objectives you should be working towards in the next year.
- Considering what development or training you need to improve or enable further development.
- Considering your potential for promotion or taking on different levels or types of responsibility..

At the appraisal meeting it is important that each view is shared and that a personal development plan is prepared.

Personal development plan (PDP)

This is a plan which specifies your learning and development needs and targets for improving your job performance. Components of a PDP are:

- clear objectives
- a range of activities under headings such as job activities, work-based learning, projects, education, training and experiences etc
- contingency plans if there are any barriers to progress
- performance measures to determine success
- ways of reviewing and dates for review.

Be prepared to review your plan on a frequent basis your circumstances or those within your workplace may change, learning opportunities may no longer be available or more appropriate ones may come along. It is also essential that the plan takes account of your personal needs as well as your professional needs. There must be a balance between your home and working life. The following opportunities may help you achieve your plan.

Exploiting opportunities

Most organisations offer many opportunities for development. Although universities' accredited courses are important, there are a lot of other valuable ways of learning and developing.

Work-based learning

- Supervised practice: being supervised by a more experienced nurse will help to identify strengths and weaknesses.
- Observation: of others will help you to learn different ways of doing things and identify good practices that you will wish to follow.
- Projects: volunteering to develop patient information materials, undertake patient surveys or help to develop a ward or department policy will provide opportunities to develop new skills and will show others you are willing and interested in wider patient care activities.
- Keeping a reflective diary: will help you learn from events in your practice.
- Taking on additional responsibilities: many hospitals use link or key nurse systems to ensure good practices are disseminated, for example in tissue viability, palliative care, health and safety and for training. Investment is made in training link nurses and providing them with information to pass on to others. Acting as a link nurse has resulted in some nurses eventually becoming clinical nurse specialists.

In-house training

- Mandatory updates: most organisations require regular updates in topics such as fire safety training, CPR and manual handling.
- Clinical, management development programmes: This may be in the form of staff nurse, team leader or ward manager development programmes.
- Adhoc sessions and updates: these may be in response to new national directives, new local policies or training identified through complaints and incidents.

Post registration courses

These may be:

- clinical, management, professional, research and education or a combination
- at diploma, degree or post graduate levels.

Self development

This may be done through self directed study, reading journals, keeping a reflective diary, volunteering to be involved and joining groups within the organizations, such as journal clubs and research interest groups or within national professional bodies.

Development through support

This may be through clinical supervision, preceptorship, mentorship and action learning (*chapter 22*).

Development through experience

This may be through visiting other organisations at home or abroad, shadowing people, and undertaking secondments and study tours.

Evaluating your learning

There are two markers against which you can evaluate the effectiveness of your continuing professional development:

- Your personal development plan. Consider:
  - what progress you made against the objectives you set? In hindsight were the objectives relevant and realistic?
  - how and to what extent did the learning activities you used help you achieve your objectives? Would others have been better?
  - were there any barriers to your achieving the objectives and, if so, could you have taken any preventative measures?
  - what has been the overall impact on your ability to do your job?
- Your progress with your longer term career plan. Consider:
  - to what extent has the learning contributed to your overall career targets?
  - whether you should include any thing different in future?

Remember what you can do

- To start as you mean to go on.
- Keep your profile and portfolio up to date.
- Find out what opportunities are available in your organisation from your line manager, professional development or training department, in house magazine or notice board.
- Find out what opportunities there are outside your organisation from web sites on the internet or from professional bodies.
- Use what opportunities you can.
- Make the most of appraisals and support mechanisms that are on offer
- Reflect on your progress.

Additional reading

Edwards S (2003) Critical thinking at the bedside: a practical perspective. *Br J Nurs* **12**(19): 1142–9

Tingle J (2002) Clinical negligence and the need to keep professional updated. *Br J Nurs* **11**(20): 1304–6

Useful websites

www.britishjournalofnursing.com	British Journal of Nursing
www.internurse.com	On-line archive of peer reviewed articles
www.nursingtimes.net	Nursing Times
www.nursing-standard.co.uk	Nursing Standard
www.rcn.org.uk	Royal College of Nursing
www.nmc-uk.org	Nursing and Midwifery Council

Chapter 24

Career development

Ann Close

This chapter provides you with information on how to plan and develop your career and to identify and use the opportunities available to you. It identifies the keys to success, how to get started, make the most of opportunities and where to seek help and support from others.

What are career development and a career pathway?

Many nurses come into the profession, as they believe it will provide them with a lifelong career. This will mean different things to different people. For some it will mean seeking promotion on a planned basis from entry into the profession as a staff nurse onwards and upwards. For others it will mean developing in their role as a staff nurse as they wish to bring up a family or have other commitments or wish to combine nursing with other careers. Also it may be that they enjoy this role the best and recognise this is where they can contribute most effectively.

Some nurses will have a very clear idea of where they want their career to go and the pathway of how they are going to get there. The vast majority will not. Nowadays there are many different ways of reaching the same goal. There is no right or wrong career pathway but there are a lot of opportunities to suit every need at different times in people's lives. It is not necessary to have your end goal.

What opportunities for career development are there?

There are many opportunities available today. Whichever is chosen, continuous professional development and updating, described in chapter 23, is essential.

Staff nurses can develop their careers in a particular strand in:

- Education: in Universities or within the NHS.
- Clinical practice: as a generalist or specialist nurse or in higher level practice.
- Research: in Universities or NHS based.
- Management: in nurse management or general management.
- Professional or the Political arena: as a civil servant, trade union representative or in a professional body.
- Overseas: working in Europe, the United States or in a developing country or on a voluntary basis. (Table 24.1)

It is also possible to combine many of the above strands in joint appointments for example:

- Lecturer practitioners combining education and clinical practice.
- Clinical researchers combining clinical practice and research.
- Clinical managers combining clinical practice and management of an area.
- Education management combining education and service management or education management.

For many posts it is desirable to have experience in a few strands for example:

- In education posts it is essential to have clinical experience and useful to have research and management experience.
- For management posts it is essential to have clinical experience and useful to have research and some education experience.

The more senior the post the more advantageous it is to have a variety of experiences. For example:

- A consultant nurse requires experience as a generalist and specialist nurse and in higher level practice and have some research, management and education experiences.

Table 24.1 Career Development opportunities

Education	Clinical	Management	Research	Professional/ Politics	Overseas
Professor/ Dean	Consultant nurse	Trust level	Professor	CNO Department of Health	USA
Principle lecturer	Clinical nurse specialist	Directorate level	Reader	Head of professional body	Europe
Senior lecturer	Ward manager	Divisional of specialty level	Principle researcher	Regional level	Overseas
Lecturer	Specialist nurse	Ward manger	Research associate	Strategic Health Authority (HA) level	Voluntary services

What are the keys to success?

It essential to have a combination of the following to develop your career:

- Competencies: the skills, knowledge and capability to do what is required. These may have been learned and developed in a variety of jobs but can be transferred to new situations.
- Experience: this brings together knowledge and skills gained through learning based on actual events while working in a variety of settings.

Many nurses express a desire to work in a certain specialty on qualification and remain in that specialty for many years. This can be limiting, not only in terms of their career development but also to their ability to care holistically for patients.

Specialising early in their career may make promotion more difficult as there will be fewer posts available and often employers look for a wider experience. The vast majority of patients in hospitals have multiple pathologies and nurses with a broad base of experience usually have more understanding of all the patients' needs.

Opportunities to do rotation programmes in a variety of specialties such as six months each in medicine, surgery and critical care – will give a broad base of experience for newly registered nurses. This can then be built on by rotation through surgical specialties such as an emergency admission area, vascular surgery and surgical high dependency will give broad surgical experience to a more senior nurse who has chosen surgical nursing as a specialty.

How can I get started?

- Develop a broad base of experience: Having experience of nursing different types of patients will provide a wide range of skills and knowledge that can be transferred and used throughout your career. It will enable you to keep your options open if you are undecided on your career path.
- Experience different settings, organisations and ways of doing things. This will help to develop problem-solving skills, flexibility and a broader understanding of health care.
- Build up academic qualifications and practice experience. Academic skills help to develop an understanding of the theories that underpin practice and provide opportunities for the individual to develop practice in a structured, evidence-based way. Employers look for professionals with both the right qualifications and experience for more senior posts.
- Develop a network for information, support, advice and contacts. A network may be formal or informal and will provide access to new ideas, ways of working and broaden horizons. Networks may help to open new doors and access to new opportunities.

How can I make the most of the right opportunities and experiences?

- Keep your portfolio up to date (*Chapter 23*).
- Log experiences so that you can learn from them.
- Identify transferable skills that can be used in other situations, for example communication, project planning, negotiating, problems solving skills and many more.
- Identify achievements which will demonstrate your success in using these skills
- Use appraisal, personal development plans and all development opportunities: to further develop and refine skills and knowledge.
- Volunteer and go the extra mile. There are many opportunities, for example:
  - respond to consultation documents
  - participate in workshops on aspects of practice
  - join a working group to develop policies and guidelines
  - become a link nurse
  - prepare an information poster or leaflet for patients

- prepare a learning package for students or auxiliary nurses
- write a short piece for the in-house magazine or equivalent.

■ These will not only be useful items for your curriculum vitae but will be recognised and valued by more senior nurses and managers.

■ Be prepared to move on and 'out of the safe box': The same team of staff working together for several years tends to develop a culture and way of working that everyone becomes comfortable with and they may fail to recognise that changes are required and new ways of working are necessary. Innovation and development may be stifled and it may be necessary to move on to new experiences to stimulate continuing growth.

■ Seek guidance and get a mentor to help you discover and use your own talents.

What if I change my mind?

It may be that initially you thought you wanted to take a particular career direction but your interests or circumstances change.

■ Be positive about your current capabilities and the experiences you have had.

■ Remember the broad base of experience. This will be a much better foundation to build on than if you stayed with one specialty only.

■ Remember the transferable skills and knowledge and market them. Think carefully how they can be used in the new direction you want to take.

■ Use the networks you have developed from the beginning to access opportunities, support and advice.

■ Be prepared to move downward or sideways, if only temporarily, if it will ultimately help you to your ultimately goal.

■ Use all your experiences in the new situation.

How can I get help and support?

The key is to ASK

■ You'll never get help if you don't.

- Ask people in jobs you think you would like to do – they will be able to tell you the realities of what it is actually like and how they got the job.
- Ask to shadow or observe them – so that you can see for yourself.
- Ask for help and support at your appraisal and performance development planning meetings.
- Ask senior colleagues for advice.
- Ask your mentor.
- Ask more than one person. They will have different views and you can use these to come to your own decision.

How can I help myself?

- Be realistic about your capacity and capability. Don't take on more than you can cope with but also don't underestimate yourself.
- Remember it's your responsibility and it's down to you.
- Don't be put off.
- Be flexible and creative in your thinking.
- Reflect on experiences and learn from them.
- Try a different route if necessary to get where you want to go.

Remember what you can do

- To help and support others who are also trying to move along their career paths.
- To keep the principles and fundamentals of nursing.
- The importance of the right attitude and personality.
- Effective communication is essential to effective care.
- The importance of effective co-ordination and team working.
- To monitor and evaluate what you are doing and base your practice on evidence.
- That patients are the reason for developing your career.

Additional reading

Covey S (1992) The seven habits of highly effective people – powerful lessons in personal change. Simon Schuster, London
Davis N (2003) Access for all. *Nurs Standard* **17**(26): 96
Green H, Meehan D (2002) Planning for success. *Nurs Manag* **9**(7): 6–9
Obrey A (2002) Securing the future of the NHS. Developing and supporting staff nurses. *Nurs Manag* **9**(2): 15–7
Taylor C (2001) Be choosy. *Nurs Standard* **15**(37): 18–9

Useful websites

www.nelh.org.uk   National Electronic Library for Health
www.rcn.org.uk   Royal College of Nursing
www.nursing-standard.co.uk   Nursing Standard
www.dh.gov.uk   Department of Health

Index